A Prescription for Retail Pharmacy

A Guide to Retail Pharmacy for Patients, Doctors,
Nurses, Pharmacists, and Pharmacy Technicians

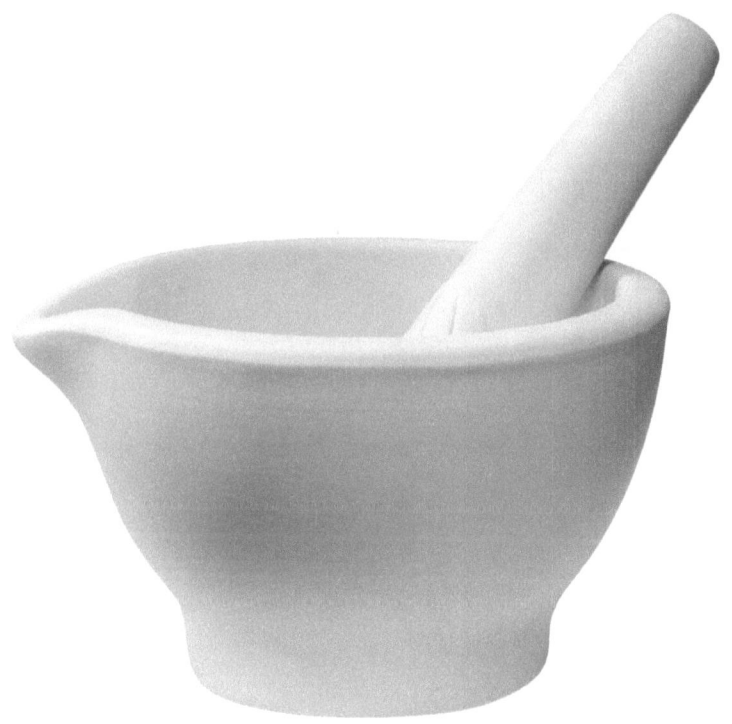

Jean-Marc Bovee, Pharm.D.

iUniverse, Inc.
Bloomington

iUniverse books may be ordered through booksellers or by contacting:

iUniverse
1663 Liberty Drive
Bloomington, IN 47403
www.iuniverse.com
1-800-Authors (1-800-288-4677)

ISBN: 978-1-4502-9484-3 (sc)
ISBN: 978-1-4502-9485-0 (hc)
ISBN: 978-1-4502-9483-6 (ebook)

Library of Congress Control Number: 2011901452

Printed in the United States of America

iUniverse rev. date: 02/15/2011

Contents

This book is dedicated to my family and friends who have endured my rants over the years, and the great Buffalo Bills of the 90's especially Don Beebe who taught me in Super Bowl XXVII to, "Never give up."

Introduction

"If Virtue and Knowledge are diffused among the People, they will never be enslav'd. This will be their great Security."

- Samuel Adams

Most books written on pharmacy are little more than academic training manuals devoid of the intimate real world interpersonal aspects involved. This book will not only serve as a guide for those who wish to understand the true inner workings of retail pharmacy, but will do so by discussing real life situations, problems, and possible solutions. The crux of this book is derived largely from my personal experiences working as a pharmacy technician (tech), and currently as a pharmacist along with contributions from friends and family who are also in the field.

I worked as a tech for five years before being accepted to pharmacy school, and earned a B.S in Biology at the University of Central Florida in the process. I then worked part-time while attending the Saint Louis College of Pharmacy (StLCoP), and graduated with my B.S. in 2002 and then my doctorate (Pharm.D.) in 2003. I also graduated as a member of the Rho Chi Pharmacy Academic Honor Society.

Over the past 18 years, I have worked for four different companies in three major cities in two separate states as either a tech or pharmacist. I have worked in at least thirty different pharmacies with dozens of different pharmacists, and even more techs, as well as under five different pharmacy supervisors. Included in my experience is six months spent as a floater pharmacist working from store to store. Despite where I work, I still face the same issues over and over again, and have been answering the exact same basic questions from customers, techs, doctors, nurses, and grocery personnel my entire career.

It is hoped that this book will aid the various aforementioned groups to navigate retail pharmacy. It will provide for better communication with retail pharmacists, serve as a guide for pharmacists to better handle various problems often encountered in the retail setting, offer suggestions for the training of techs, and make the inner workings of the retail pharmacy world common knowledge for patients. For instance, when a patient goes to see the doctor or dentist, they know what to expect. They understand the procedure they will have to endure such as the filling out of forms, the inevitable time spent in the waiting room, the continued waiting in the examination room, the eventual poking and prodding, the billing process, the follow up scheduling, etc. In short, they know the drill. Such is not yet the case in regards to retail pharmacy. I am far too often taken aback by those who still have absolutely not an inkling as to how this all works. It is time that the functioning of retail pharmacy becomes conventional wisdom.

The sheer numbers of people nationwide who still, to this day, do not understand the rigmarole involved with retail pharmacies is troublesome because our aging population will certainly escalate this need. In fact, so little progress has been made in the public's understanding of how retail pharmacies function, in the professional relationships between other medical professionals and pharmacists, and in the knowledge and training of techs that often times I feel like Bill Murray in Groundhog Day wondering when tomorrow will finally come.

It is one thing for the general public to be a bit behind, but when other health care professionals fail to get it, then the concern really kicks in. Nurses, for example, often still do not as a matter of standard procedure; spell the patient's name, the doctor's name, nor the drug when calling in a prescription (rx) on the pharmacy's voice message system (IVR). This ought to be common sense by now. What if your surgeon was this blasé'? You may have the wrong appendage amputated. Look at all we have accomplished as a species, and yet we cannot make spelling second nature in health care.

Doctors still do not understand that unless I can read their writing, and most especially their signature or DEA number, then I cannot fill the rx they have taken the time to scribble out. Rather, I have to spend half of my day tracking someone down at his or her office, or hospital, who can give me the information that I require. As time goes on, because of the increasing scarce remnants of a good work ethic and competency among our workforce, this task becomes harder and takes longer to accomplish.

This book is also intended to spark a movement at the state level at least, and the federal level at best, to develop certain much needed laws; laws that should have been passed eons ago. For instance, laws on penmanship should be much more wide spread, and the ones on the books now need to be better enforced. We have such laws in Florida, but most everyone seems completely oblivious to them. Doctors ought to consider what their neglect could lead to.

A law requiring standardization of tech training and licensing is long past due. Soon registration will be mandatory in many states, but as I write this, only ten states require certification. Techs are intimately involved in patient care. They type rxs, handle phone calls, grab the bottles off of the shelves, count or measure the quantity of the drugs, and ultimately dispense the medicine directly to the patients. Unfortunately, the average tech is dangerously unqualified, and when I say 'dangerously' I mean exactly that.

In most states, anyone on the street can apply and get a job as a tech. All that is required is a nametag that says "Pharmacy

Technician." This is not the case for the ancillary staff in any other branch of medicine. Some techs are apathetic and have no desire to be competent, and some simply lack the ability. Then there are others who take a little from column A, and a little from column B. In fact, it is so rare to find a good tech that pharmacists will fight to get them into their store with the same vehemence that Dr. Jones chased after the Lost Ark.

There is no formal education required, and there are very few standardized training programs. Basically, it is up to every company to develop their own system. Some use training manuals and instructional CDs, some use trainers, and some simply allow the pharmacist at a particular store to handle the training. Pharmacy supervisors are seldom helpful for they wish not to be bothered with issues of micro-management. Obviously, this leaves a vast variety of ability from company to company, pharmacy to pharmacy, and tech to tech.

Regardless, it all spells disaster for pharmacists who cherish their license, for companies that would rather not be sued for millions of dollars, and especially patients whose lives are at stake, literally. It is a testament to pharmacists everywhere that the number of patients who die each year from medication errors, or Quality Related Events (QREs), does not number into the tens of thousands.

When all is said and done, hopefully there will be more homogeneity between techs, better communication and relations between pharmacists and other health care professionals, and a better understanding among retail pharmacy patients. This will not only make pharmacists' jobs easier, but will allow the entire medical system to function more efficiently. It will also provide more and better safety, comfort, and service for the general public. As our population ages, the need to better understand retail pharmacy grows more critical. This book will help to navigate the constantly changing and increasingly complex world of retail pharmacy.

Other questions will hopefully be answered as well such as: Why do doctors write in hieroglyphics? Why do they allow receptionists to not only call in rxs to pharmacies posing as nurses, but to also pose as physician assistants and approve drugs or dosages without their knowledge? Why don't nurses spell? Why are the techs with the most experience the worst ones? How does a pharmacist determine how long it will take to fill a rx? What do you tell an obvious drug addict who is asking for syringes? How do you deal with and remove a bad apple from your pharmacy? What do pharmacy supervisors do exactly? What does the future hold for retail pharmacy? I will try to answer these questions, and more. Like Benjamin Franklin said, "Human felicity is produc'd not so much by great pieces of good fortune that seldom happen, as by little advantages that occur every day."

Advice for Patients

"He that won't be counseled can't be helped."

– Benjamin Franklin

Are you ready folks? Here's how it works: you drop off a rx and your prescription insurance card (not your medical or dental card). Then you go away for a while, while we type it up. Our computer electronically sends the rx to your insurance company's computer, your insurance company's computer sends the price that we are supposed to charge you to our printer, and then we physically fill the rx. When you come back you are charged whatever your insurance company told us to charge you. Simple enough concept, eh? Then why is it that, to this day, the vast majority of people still do not understand this? (Appendix A)

Due to the aforementioned in depth explanation, I trust there will be no more questions about cost while dropping the rx off at the window, right? Well, there ought not be, anyway. We do not know the price of your rx until we fill it under your insurance first. All we can do before filling it is to provide the cash price. Now you finally know why that is. I am sincerely sorry that no one has ever explained that to you previous to the publication of this book.

In point of fact, in January 2010 a 90-year-old man actually dropped off two rxs and flat out asked me, "How does this work?" I thought to myself, "Good for him for finally asking." It is lamentable, however, that no one ever took the relatively brief time to explain this to him anytime during the last century. Unfortunately, some customers, even after your dissertation, will still argue with you claiming that it does not work that way, in fact. Then you want to ask them, "Have you ever worked in a pharmacy? No? Then how in the hell would you know? Why would I make up such an explanation? Why don't you take my word for it? What's the debate about?"

Questions like, "Why is it so much?" or comments like, "It didn't cost that much before!" are grating after a while as well. We do not know why the charge is what it is, or why it has changed. We can only speculate. It is best if you call your insurance and ask them yourself. Things do tend to go up in cost over time, and drugs are no exception. "I don't remember paying that much for it before! Did the price go up from last month?" We do not know off hand. You can't remember what you paid, but you expect me too? Sure, we can look it up for you, but why not just ask for that in the first place before yelling at us?

If it was less before, then it is safe to say that the price has gone up, isn't it? Maybe your deductible has rolled over. Maybe the drug's tier has changed. Also, if you get a new card, please give it to us at the same time that you drop off your rx. If you wait until pick up, then you are only delaying the process because now we have to go back to square one.

"Why isn't this drug covered?!" Again, only your insurance company knows the answer to that question. See that 1-800 number on the back of your insurance card titled "Customer Service?" I could call them for you, but if I had to do that for everyone who questioned their co-pay, then I'd never get anything else done. It takes a mighty long time to get a human being on the phone. "Press one if you are calling from the continental U.S. Press two if you are calling from Guatemala. Press three if you are calling from south of the equator." I'm sorry, but this is one area where patients need to take a more active roll in their own health care. We are a pharmacy, not an insurance agency. Besides, you had to have received a packet from your prescription insurance company at some point explaining what drugs are covered, what tiers they are on, and what your various co-pays will be.

I particularly like it when they say, "It should be the same amount I paid last time." My typical reply is, "But apparently it's not, and wouldn't be if the price has gone up now would it?" Then they try to flank you by pleading, "Can't you just give it to me for what it was last time?" To which I respond, "Well, um, wait...let me think about that for a seco...NO." Do you realize that, in essence, what you are asking is that we pay for part of your co-pay?

Now for a few loose ends. Your prescription insurance card is wholly different most of the time from your medical or dental card. It usually has an "Rx" on it somewhere, and a "BIN" number, which is sort of like the insurance card's ID number. This is not always the case, of course. Sometimes one card does it all, but rarely. By the way, this will be the only instance in this book where I will take the time to point out that exceptions obviously exist whenever generalizations occur. Got that?

In any case, you signed these contracts when you chose them, so if you have done your homework, then you should know which of your cards are for what, and how much your co-pay ought to be. After all, this is your health and money we are talking about here. If your insurance rejects your rx, and you want us to call them to find out why, then that is fine, we are happy to help, but it will take time. Please do not stand there glaring at me holding up the line expecting immediate resolution. Oh, and staring does not expedite anything. In fact, I periodically have to tell my customers that, "My concentration suffers greatly when I am observed."

Not only does it take a lot of number punching to get an insurance representative on the phone, but we also have many other sick people requiring our immediate help (i.e., we suffer from constant interruptions). Sometimes we do not have time to make an instant phone call. It is much easier for everyone if you call your insurance yourself, but if you prefer, then we will do it, and then we will call you when the mystery has been solved. If you do not hear from us in a day or two, then you are more than welcome to call us back and inquire about your rx.

Hopefully you did not wait until you were completely out of pills before you dropped off your refill (ahem). If that is the case, we will certainly give you a few pills to get you by until the matter has been settled, unless it is a controlled drug or something that cannot be partially filled such as an inhaler. In these cases it is that particular pharmacist's judgment call. Again, as a single person, it is easier for you to follow up with us once ample time has passed.

The same goes for doctor calls. Often times someone drops off their rx bottle for a refill, and it either has no refills left or is expired (both of which are indicated right on the rx vial itself). So then we are ordered, I mean asked, to call the doctor's office for another rx. As the patient walks toward the ice cream section with their grocery cart I have to say to them, "You do realize this will take time." The response is usually something like, "Oh, that's okay, I have some shopping to do. What do you think, ten minutes?" I absolutely love it when customers tell me what the wait time is going to be. Giggling, I typically reply, "No, when I say time I mean 24 to 48 hours." Then I get that look. It is the look of the vengeful warrior that every pharmacist can recognize.

I mean honestly, would you prefer we provide you the number you wish to hear, or the more probable and realistic one? I can tell you it will be ready in seven seconds if you want. Listen, I'll cross my fingers and hope that your doctor calls me back in the next few minutes, but I will not hold my breath. Once he or she calls I will fill your rx as fast as humanly possible, but I can't do any better than that.

It is not we pharmacists who set the time frame, just as it is not we who set your co-pay. We are simply giving you a realistic assessment of when your doctor will get back to us. Think of us as the monkey in the middle. We simply do as we're told by the physician, and the insurance company. We are the Rodney Dangerfield of the medical professions. Helpful hint: the doctor's office will probably approve your refills a lot sooner if they hear from you as well.

Whenever we call your doctor's office, for whatever reason, we often get a machine which states, "Please provide for 24 to 48 hours for a response," and then allows us to leave a message. Have you ever tried to get a hold of your doctor right away? I rest my case.

Once I have beat this drum long enough, made my point, and the patient realizes the situation, then they always ask me, "Well, once it is approved can you call me?" Sure, in the name of customer service I'd be happy to, but again we have a hundred calls to make every day, you have one. A lot also depends on how busy we are that day, if our tech calls in sick, and many other unpredictable factors. Again, if you do not hear from us within a few hours, then check back later in the day, and we will gladly give you the current status of your rx.

All we ask is that you please do not harass us every hour on the hour. That is the number one cause of eye twitching in a retail pharmacy setting. My right eyelid spasses out so fast sometimes, that hummingbirds fluttering nearby often times try to mate with it.

"But I need it now! I am out!" Okay, so you are waiting to the last minute to get the medication that keeps you alive, and this is our fault? It seems that thinking ahead in anticipation of something possibly going wrong is a lost consideration these days.

Fine, we will make the effort when we have the time, but believe it or not, a lot of pharmacies are so damn busy that they literally don't have the time; they really do not. This is especially more the case nowadays since companies are cutting back on tech help for pharmacists, and forcing us to give flu shots, among other things. Let's all work together for your benefit. Do not be afraid to be an active player in your own health care, and remember, don't shoot the messenger.

I once had a woman call for a drug that we did not have, so she wanted me to call pharmacies all around town and try to find it for her. I explained I would when I had time, but was unsure when that would be, and that it may be quicker for her to grab a phone book and call the stores closest to her location. "Oh, but I am very sick. I can't do it." She called me three times that afternoon checking to see if I had found it for her yet. I was scratching my head; clearly she could make these calls herself.

Usually I'll call a couple of pharmacies, but if no one has the drug, then what am I to do? Am I to call ten, twenty, fifty pharmacies? No, at some point you need to chip in and grab the baton; after all, it is your health we're talking about here.

As I have come to learn, it is much easier for people to ask someone else rather than to get the answer themselves. Pharmacists and techs are no exception to this. I have worked with people who often blurt out, "Where's the rx for so-and-so?" Then I say, "All you have to do is hit F3, type in the patient's last name, and the computer will tell you which queue it is in." Of course, this exact same exchange is repeated multiple times throughout the day.

Often a customer will walk right up to me and ask, "Where are your cough drops?" Then I say, "Look down and reach out," all the while thinking, "If you had taken one millisecond to look around you would have seen the item you're looking for, and would not have had to interrupt me and break my concentration."

Also, why debate us? This may sound like a pretentious question, but we do not tell anyone anything that is not as it is. When the price prints out, don't yell at us-it is what it is. When your drug is not covered by your insurance, don't argue with us-it is what it is. If we do not have the drug in stock, don't get mad at us personally, we did not do it on purpose, I swear. And why are you mad at me because your doctor has not approved our refill request for you yet? We called him, and we faxed his office. What have you done? Have you tried to contact him yourself yet? Well, why not? Why leave it solely to us? It's your health, how about some participation? They may be able to ignore us, they hear from pharmacies all day long, but it is harder for them to ignore the patient once they call. I mean seriously, what do you want me to do, go over to the doctor's office and put him in a head lock?

Often times, the patient will say, "I'm here to pick up a rx. My doctor's office called it in." After a thorough search I respond, "No, I'm sorry, I don't see anything." Then the patient exclaims, "The doctor said he called it in," or "I saw him fax it." Then I'll say, "Are you sure they called (or faxed) the correct pharmacy?" Invariably the response is "Yes! I gave them your number." Then, after a second exhaustive search, I say, "I'm sorry. I don't have it. They must not have done it yet." What follows in a minor temper tantrum directed at the pharmacy staff.

Now, what are you people thinking? It is almost as if customers assume I'm joking with them, that I am hiding the rx behind my back, and at any minute I'll pull it out and say, "Okay, just kidding, I had it right here the whole time. You got me. I was just messing with you." Listen, if we say we do not have the rx, then it is because we do not have it yet. We are not magicians who can pull your rx out of our butt, and it is not our fault the doctor's office has failed to send it to us.

Please do not haggle with us on your wait time either. Do you honestly think we arbitrarily make up those minutes? We say it will take a half an hour because we want to make sure it will be ready when you get back so that you do not bark at us if it is not. It may only take twenty minutes, but we cannot guarantee it vis-à-vis interruptions, problems, issues, etc. so we say thirty instead just to cover our rear end.

It is what it is. Get the idea? Besides, rushing leads to errors. In a perfect world you would not have to wait at all. Also, I think I speak for all pharmacists when I say that we are tired of hearing about your melting ice cream. Of all the things we have to worry about, your melting ice cream is about 8 billionth on the list.

Now this is important, when I ask you for your "last name" please don't say your entire name. About one thousand times throughout my career I have asked a customer, who is picking up their rx, "What is your last name?" Then I hear, "Miranda Conchita Alanzo Lopez Rodriguez." See, when you do that I don't know where to start looking. I'll probably begin searching in the "M's." Please, when I ask for the last name, just say your **last** name. Along those lines, if I ask you to spell your last name, then do not simply re-pronounce it. There is a difference between spelling and pronouncing, okay?

Also, what is the deal with patients dangling their rxs just out of our reach when we lean over the counter to grab them? Exactly how long must we remain in these uncomfortable and ridiculous positions before you deem us worthy to take your ever so deeply valued rxs away from you? Sometimes it feels like patients are dropping their kids off at summer camp such is the strength of the apparent attachment to them. Perhaps it is the realization that they will never see these rxs again once they hand them over, but then you have to wonder how such a bond could develop after a short drive from the doctor's office to the pharmacy. Listen people, just hand us the friggin' scripts already.

One thing I thought would be common knowledge by now is that a rx is only good for one year, unless it is a controlled drug, then it is six months. All too often a confrontation ensues when a customer calls in for a refill, we see that it is expired, we state that we have to call the doctor for a new rx, the patient yells that they still have several refills, and finally we explain that it could have 100 refills but that is irrelevant if the rx itself is expired.

An entire book could be written about the various types of patients out there, and the experiences I've had with them over the years. For instance, you have the insouciant curmudgeon whose life is obviously full of much rage and free time. This chronically unpleasant person's colonic sphincter is strung so tight, that you can smell the bile on their breath as they chastise you for some minor indiscretion you committed. There is no pleasing this person, and if you stumble just a tad, then they will devote their empty lives to making as many phone calls and writing as many letters that they can to your peers and superiors in an effort to get you fired. Jihadists marvel at the vindictiveness of these people especially when one considers how little it took to set them off in the first place. You can imagine how much fun we Florida pharmacists have with snowbirds in this regard. In the appendix is an article that I was able to get published in a local newspaper on the subject. (Appendix B)

However, that is not what this chapter is about. Patients need advice on how to deal with pharmacists, and ultimately this will benefit everyone involved. There are just a few rules one has to remember.

Rule number one is to be patient (no pun intended). Even if you are in a hurry, you have to realize that so are a lot of other patients as well, even if you do not see them. They have dropped off their rx, and are now shopping around soon to be back. Rushing the pharmacist is not a good idea. The more we rush, the more we open the floodgates to mistakes. Lastly, in this regard, do not tell us you are going on vacation and have a plane to catch unless it is the literal truth because this line is used so often that we simply cannot believe so many people could coincidentally be vacationing all at once. I think I can speak for most retail pharmacists in the country when I say that we are not buying that line anymore. The fabric of our society would collapse if every person who said they were going on vacation were actually doing so. Maybe if we were in Europe it would be more believable.

The second rule is do not stare. If we say it will be 15 minutes or so, then go walk around, or have a seat. Standing there and staring at us through the window is not going to make us work any faster, and may, in fact, have the opposite effect if the pharmacist working on your rx gets ticked off enough. Here's a news flash- you are not our only customer. Also, rudeness will get you nowhere. You cannot be rude and expect results. Did you get that New Yorkers? Also, I will ring up a few grocery items for you, but when you pull up with a grocery cart filled to the brim, then you have gone too far. We have to draw the line somewhere. When I was a tech our policy was three items or less. Once I had a guy with about a dozen items say, "Well, just ring me up four different times." I wanted to say, "You're sort of missing the point jerk." Voltaire said it best, "Common sense is not so common."

Third rule is please do not yell at us. When I tell my friends and family, who are not members of the retail pharmacy world, daily anecdotes about my customers they are dumfounded as to how someone could be so rude and confrontational to a total stranger; especially a stranger with an advanced medical degree. Think about it before you go off on us, we are trying to help you.

Listen, we want to give you your medicine; we have no reason not to. However, for a variety of reasons, something may come up and we cannot readily fill your rx. Honestly, we are trained health care professionals, not shoe salespeople like Al Bundy. There is no reason to fly off of the handle. You do not even know us. To be so impolite and disrespectful to a perfect stranger is to have no decorum whatsoever. Would you treat your doctor this way, or a perfect stranger passing you on the street for that matter? C'mon, it's not like we're making Happy Meals back here. This isn't McPills, all right?

Many times, a patient will come to their senses, after the problem has been resolved, and will say, "I'm sorry for being so rude. I know it's not your fault." Just once I want to rub it in and ask indignantly, "Then why were you yelling at me? Something doesn't go as you planned, and that's an excuse for freaking out?" It's not a perfect world, stuff happens. Why on earth wouldn't we fill this rx as soon as possible, and get you out the door? You know, I could run over my dog in the driveway on the way to work, my kid could break her arm on the playground at school, and my wife could get fired, and I still would not treat a total stranger with that degree of contempt over such relative frivolities.

Like when your prescription insurance drops the ball, why take it out on us? Do you yell at your plumber because the air conditioner isn't working? How about your mailman because the lawn guy hasn't cut your grass yet? So why shout in my face about your insurance? We have little or no say in what your insurance does, honestly.

Rule number four, please do not just walk up without any specifics, or anything in hand and simply say things like, "I need a prescription." My response will be, "What luck, I happen to dispense prescriptions!" If you reply, "I need a refill," then I will ask you what the name of the medication is. Often, at this point, the usual response is, "I can't remember." C'mon people, use your head and get in the game.

Especially you middle aged baby boomers, you're old enough by now. You cannot remember the name of the drug that keeps your eyes from bleeding? How is that possible?! Seriously, you may not be so old that you remember when the wonder drugs of the day were camphor and castor oil, but I know you must have frequented a retail pharmacy before at some point. Again, here is a prime example of someone not getting his or her game face on. Please help us to help you. I get more phone calls where the person says, "I need to refill my Diovan®." Then, after an exceedingly long pause, I actually have to say, "And your name is.......?"

Speaking of wonder drugs, do you know why they are called that? Because you have to wonder if they will work, as opposed to a miracle drug which is thus called because it's any medicine you can get a child to take without screaming. That is my pharmacy humor. Anyway...

Fellow pharmacists, ever notice how irritated people get when you don't know them? People, I understand you have been coming to this pharmacy for a while now, but I am new here. Have you ever seen me before? Lemme cover up my name badge...okay what is my name? There are hundreds of you and only one of me. Get it? Lighten up.

Rule five, please try to pay attention at all times. On a daily basis at least one patient gets mad at us for our hours. "I was here at eight this morning but you don't open until nine!" All I can muster in response is, "True." Usually they get angriest about our lunch hours, "I didn't know you closed a half an hour for lunch. I've been sitting here for 30 minutes!" Whenever someone expresses irateness because we were closed when they showed up I poignantly point out that our hours are clearly posted, and have been since the store was erected, as they are in **every** pharmacy.

Seriously, what do you expect us to do, apologize for your ignorance? Perhaps we ought to have a flashing, voice activated, red neon sign that announces our hours on a continuous loop (kind of like the 'Walk/Don't Walk" street signs in Blade Runner). Attentiveness will also help you decipher between the pick up and drop off windows. The cash register is a big clue. A minimally attentive person will see that, and hopefully deduce that the pick up window is probably there.

Having your wits about you will also prevent hair-pulling conversations like the following one that I had with a customer while I was ringing him up. I asked him, "Do you have prescription insurance?" His simple reply was, "No." After I scan his four rxs he inquires, "Did my insurance not cover any of it?" Hesitantly I respond, "When I just asked you if you have insurance your answer was 'No,' so where did I lose you?" "Oh no, I have insurance, I'm sorry."

Addendum to rule five involves paying attention to the instructions on the signature capture device as you pay at the register. Now, I know every place has a different machine with different directions. Sometimes you swipe it this way, sometimes that way...I understand, but this is not a detonator, okay? You do not need a flow chart or a schematic diagram to figure it out. All you have to do is be able to see, read, follow simple directions, and then push the appropriate buttons. Blind people have pet monkeys that can do all of that. Some of you act like you're disarming a bomb. Sweat is dripping off of the brow, that intense look in the eyes, the painstaking eye to hand movements...look, just press enter! I am reminded of the scene in Zoolander where Ben Stiller and Owen Wilson are beating on the computer like Kubrick apes. It is 2011, and you are still unfamiliar with the present day payment process? You're making George H. W. Bush look like Steve Freakin' Jobs!

This is especially true when you ask me, "Where do I sign?" I want you to just think about the words "signature capture" for a second. How about on the line that says "signature?"

When you sign your name, it is okay to simply initial. A lot of times it seems people are signing their Lord of the Ring name- Sarah Jessica Bungee Cord Smith-Jones of Bunghole Gardens, Daughter of Edgar from Stinks Ville, protector of the helpless, surveyor of the measureless....blah, blah, blah. Lady! Just sign your damn name already, okay?! What in the world is taking so long? Right behind her is Apollo Creed, Master of Disaster, the King of Sting, the Count of Monte Fisto....come on people! Just put a damn "X" for all I care, but let's get a move on! It didn't take Madison and Hamilton that long to write the freaking Federalist Papers, or for Jefferson to churn out the Declaration of Independence for crissakes.

Few things are as annoying than for the pharmacist to be standing there while you try to figure out how to pay, you're punching buttons like a madman, beeping sounds are going off like crazy, and then at some point you begin staring at us as if to say, "Now what?" So then we look over, and in blinking words the device says, "Please slide card." That's when my eyes roll over to the back of my skull, an aura comes over me along with a sharp stabbing pain square in my cranium, and I begin to wonder what the hell you have been doing for the last two and a half minutes. What did you think was going on? What did you think that beeping sound was all about? And what buttons were you pushing anyway? Did you at any point actually read what the damn thing was saying? What was it Nietzsche said about herd animals?

Rule six, get off of your cell phone before approaching us. The HIPPA laws prohibit us from discussing your medication with you when someone else may overhear. Oh yeah, and it is also remarkably rude.

Many times a patient will call their doctor's office after we inform them that we have yet to hear back regarding their refill request. Invariably, they try to hand us their cell phone once they get a hold of the nurse so that we may take the rx over their phone. Sorry, but this is inappropriate and unprofessional. Tell your doctor's nurse, or assistant, to call us on our phone. I am not going to subject my self to the Ebola virus just because one of my impatient patient's insists that I immediately take the call from their cell phone. No offense.

Just as annoying as the cell phone customer is the one who walks up to the pharmacy yelling, "Hello?! Hello?!" before they're even at the counter yet. Sheez! Give it a couple of seconds, and if I don't see you, then say, "Excuse me," or something. These are probably the same people I lovingly refer to as "drive-by garbage shooters." Periodically you come to work only to find empty plates and utensils left by some customer who got them from the lady handing out samples in the deli department. Rather than dispose of their trash in one of the thirteen garbage cans strategically placed all around the store, they place it right on your pharmacy counter.

Sometimes it seems as if customers expect me to be Arnold Swarzenegger in Terminator 2 stoically standing at the counter constantly on guard, with my mortar and pestle in hand, staring out the window hours on end just waiting for someone to come. Or perhaps they expect me to be like the guard at the Tomb of the Unknown Soldier just pacing back and forth waiting for customers to walk up to my counter. Maybe we are busy at the moment you approach the counter, maybe our back is turned and we don't see you right away, maybe we just gave gas and had to pause for a nanosecond. I'm not going to immediately drop what I am doing just because you do not want to wait one moment longer than necessary. We will not be breaking any Guinness records today, sorry.

Another thing, all retail pharmacies fill generic automatically if it is available, so there is no need to ask us to do so. What you do have to mention is if you prefer the brand name drug. Now, a lot of controversy surrounds generic versus brand name drugs. For 98% of medications, the generic is the same damn thing. There are exceptions, but very few. When you pay five times more for brand, all you are doing is paying for the patent, research, studying, and marketing that went into it, which amounts to about $1 billion per drug. The manufacturers that supply the generic do not have to get back that investment. This is why they can charge so much less. It is not because generic is not as good or pure. Unlike in the lay world, generic does not equal inferior in pharmacy.

Also, every drug has a generic name given to it when it is invented. Often a patient will see that their drug has a generic name, and then indignantly ask, "Why wasn't this filled generic?" It is because there is no generic for your drug in the marketplace yet. It takes seven years before the patent runs out. If the producer of it can find a new indication for the drug, then you have to wait years longer. "But it says the generic name right here!" "Ugh, were you not listening?" This discussion is one of those that can go round and round like an Abbott and Costello Who's On First routine, or for you youngsters out there, Jerome and Morris Day trying to come up with a password.

Sometimes people get mad at us for having a mystery rx insurance card on file for them insisting that they have had only one insurance plan since wooly mammoths roamed the earth. Listen, we do not just go around adding insurance policies to people's profiles, just like we do not randomly refill rxs. You must have given us this insurance card at some point just as you must have called in that refill that you insist should not have been filled. We do not do things for no reason. Trust me on this one.

Oh, and when your doctor calls in a rx for you on our IVR do not come by three minutes later expecting it to be ready. These messages do not pop up immediately despite the fact that every doctor thinks their rx is "high priority." There is a delay between the time the call was made and when it shows up on our monitor, and besides, we may be too busy to get to it even after it pops up. Just because the M.D. called it in five minutes ago does not mean it was ready four minutes ago, or that it will be ready even an hour from now. It all depends on how busy we are at the time. The same goes for when you call in your refills.

Lastly, please do not wait until the last minute to pick up or drop off your rx. I swear, I am busier during the last 15 minutes of every shift than at any other time during my twelve-hour day. Studies show that a full one-third of Americans on unemployment find a job within 30 days after their benefits run out. Why is that I wonder? Could it be because we are a bunch of procrastinators? I can see my customers sitting on the couch in front of the TV noticing the time and saying to themselves, "Oh my gosh! The pharmacy closes in 15 minutes, I had better hurry and go drop off my rx!" Please don't do that. Otherwise you may hear your pharmacist say, "Okay, it will be ready tomorrow. You can pick it up in the morning." You see, we just spent 12 hours in this tiny little room with a limited menu, and very few bathroom breaks. We are tired and want to go home now.

One final request, it seems there is a massive conspiracy out there run by some organization that constantly surveils pharmacists. The Crips, the Bloods, MS13, Jihadists, PETA, etc. are not nearly as efficient at pulling off their sinister plots. The goal of this particular diabolical organization is to harass pharmacists. For instance, they alert their operatives as soon as the tech goes on break, and once they receive this intel, then, posed as patients with rxs, they come-a-runnin'. Like clockwork, as soon as your help is gone, people start showing up in droves. This fiendish group will also wait to see when you are preparing your lunch or dinner, then, just as you're about to eat, the gang attacks, "He's about to bite down people! Go! Go! Go!" Seriously, the consistency of this phenomenon is absolutely unbelievable. If you have any information regarding this gang of annoyers, then, for the love of God, please contact your nearest pharmacist.

Common Customer Queries

"I was gratified to be able to answer properly. I said I don't know."

- Mark Twain

Anyone who has seen Clerks or Don't Shoot the Pharmacist knows how annoying working any retail job can be. In Clerks there is a collage of dumb customer questions and comments, which I can say from first hand experience are not exaggerated. The most relatable scene was the one where a girl asks about the price of something, and right behind her is a massive sign with arrows answering her question. People do not want to read signs, even if it only consists of three words such as, "Closed for lunch."

I once worked for a company where periodically I would stay in the pharmacy during my lunch break, but I still closed the blinds, locked the door, and turned out the lights. I then would try to rest and relax for half an hour. More than once I was startled by someone who absolutely could not see me, but nonetheless was knocking on the door and windows in an attempt to get some customer service. This monolithic pearl of cluelessness, this diamond studded dimwit positively did not realize we were closed for lunch despite the signs, and thought to herself, "Well, if I continue to knock on this seemingly abandoned pharmacy, someone is sure to help me sooner or later. The windows are closed, the door is locked, and the lights are off, but someone must surely be in there." I never got a good look at their faces, but I wondered sometimes if they were just one of our Down Syndrome patients, or in this case Way Down Syndrome.

There was one day, shortly after I graduated, when we had some nurses set up a table in the store for administering flu shots. The people would walk right in, and head straight to the pharmacy to ask where the table was set up. After having enough of the interruptions, my tech and I decided to make a sign explaining where the shots were being administered. People ignored the sign and continued to interrupt us with their query. So we doubled the size of the sign, and put it directly in front of our window. They looked right over it, and continued bugging us as the sign sat silently at their chin. Disgruntled now, we decided to actually hang it from a string dead center in our pharmacy window where they would not even be able to see us without having to move it.

What happened next is pharmacy folklore in our area. They would, in fact, push the hanging sign aside and ask us, "Where are you giving the flu shots?" We were befuddled. My tech and I looked at each other with a morose melancholy that one only gets when they come to the realization that all hope is lost. I imagine the captain of the Titanic or Col. Custer had just that sort of look on their face before their sinking, or scalping. It is hard to describe the feeling. It makes you want to join Alcoholics Unanimous. You just know that it is hopeless, and there is absolutely nothing anyone can do. You're not sure what the future holds for the human race, you just hope that you won't be around to see it.

Anyway, following is a list of some of the more stupid questions and comments I have received in retail pharmacy over the years:

1. "Why do I have to fill out the patient info sheet?"

2. "Do I really have to wait 10 minutes?"

3. "I don't know the name of the doctor I saw."

4. "Where's the bathroom?" or "Where do you keep the razor blades?"

5. "Why are you out of this drug? Don't u keep it in stock?" (Well, apparently not, or it would be here wouldn't it?)

6. "What do you mean it's not ready?"

7. "I need this now. I have a plane to catch." (rx written 3 months ago)

8. "I'm from out-of-state and forgot my medication." (most New Jerseyites)

9. "Can you tell me what it will cost under my insurance before you fill it?"

10. "What do you mean my insurance won't pay for it? What, the drug?"

11. "They did it for me here *before!*" or "It wasn't that much *before!*"

12. "How come your pharmacy doesn't have a drop box for rxs?"

13. "What is this drug for?" (Why did you see the Dr. in the first place?)

14. "My grandmother (or dog) needs some syringes."

15. "Why are you out of ice cream?"

16. "Do you have any Fruit Roll-Ups without Spider Man on them?"

17. "Why don't they make this 100 count bottle in 120 count size?"

18. "What color are the tablets inside?" (Sorry, I don't have x-ray vision.)

19. "Do you carry piñatas?"

20. "Why is there no charge?" "Because it is one of our free antibiotics." "But *why* is it free?"

Honorable mention:

All too often, people go to the drop off window trying to pick up their rx, and go to the pick up window trying to drop it off. While this is mildly annoying, what is worse is when they come to the pick up window to pay for their rx, and then hand you their insurance card. No, no, see we need that beforehand. Now we have to page a grocery manager to come and void the rx out of the pharmacy register, enter the insurance card into the computer, transmit the claim to your insurance company, and then start all over again at the pick up window. If you do not hand us your insurance card at the same time you drop off the rx, then you are going to be waiting much longer than you would otherwise.

The crème de la crème of profoundly stupid requests was one provided by my wife. Apparently a woman came in to her pharmacy and asked that her narcotic rx be transferred from one Walgreens to another Walgreens. Just one problem, my wife does not work for Walgreens. Think about that for a second, let it settle, and then move on. She also had a customer call in a refill, and then expect to be able to pick it up at a pharmacy in another state! These people are true mouth-breathers. You know, the kind of person who would not be able to find his or her own bellybutton with a funnel. You can see right through their empty eyes straight to the back of their head.

If you work anywhere near an airport, then you very often have many foreign travelers coming in who ask questions like where the deutchenfrapin cream is. I will then ask them where they are from, and when they answer, I tell them that that is where it is. Then they get mad at you because in their country it is over-the-counter and no rx is necessary. "Well, welcome to America, Hans!" Really now, what is the point of that comment? Obviously we are not in your dumb country now are we?

It is tough trying to communicate with someone who speaks little or no English. Florida is the poster child for this. Hispanic patients become positively indignant when you tell them you do not speak Spanish. No seriously, they get ticked off at you. I actually had one woman's granddaughter tell me through translation that I ought to learn Spanish. When I asked why, her grandmother apparently said, "Because so many of them are coming here now." That's nice, isn't it? This also happened to a friend of mine who is a pharmacist in Orlando.

I could not believe it. Here was an elderly Hispanic woman on U.S. tax payer funded Medicaid telling me that I should learn her language admittedly because of the invasion of illegal immigrants currently underway. If they were all legal, then we would not be so overrun, and assimilation would be more likely.

So if China happened to be south of our border and they disrespected our laws and national sovereignty, then would we have to have everything printed in half Chinese too? With their fancy little symbols? My Chinese/Vietnamese wife is a pharmacist as well so when a Hispanic person asks her if she speaks Spanish she replies, "No. Do you speak Cantonese?" She becomes especially indignant because she came here and learned the language in six months, "...so why can't they?" Simple, there is no incentive to assimilate because we cater to them to such a degree. I once wrote an article about working retail pharmacy in Florida for one of my pharmacy school classes, which raised the professor's eyebrows to say the least. When approached about it I told her, "Don't worry, I'm an equal opportunity pisser-offer." For more on this subject matter please see the appendix. (Appendix C)

While we're on the subject of Hispanics may I make a humble request? Spanish people- please pick a last name and date of birth, and stick with it. I do not quite understand this, but Latinos have multiple last names, and dates of birth. Often when they pick up their rx I ask, "And what is your last name?" I then would get something like, "Ortega." When I cannot find any filled rxs under that name I ask again for clarification, but this time the answer is, "Rodriguez." We then have "Sanchez", "Gonzales", and "Vega." Eventually it gets resolved, but it sure would make things much easier if they had one last name.

I once had a gray haired Hispanic man with a date of birth that made him 22 years of age. He clearly was not a day under 50. Now, I don't want to be cynical here, but I have read much about people milking the welfare system with fake social security numbers as well as forged birth certificates. I am convinced that this has much to do with what I am describing here.

In Florida you get a lot of, "You speaka Espanol?" My reply to this is, "No. You speaka English?" They'll say no and then stare at you like their language is just going to come to you through divine inspiration. There are many things I wish I could say to these people like, "This is North America not South or Central America, do you think it may be a good idea to learn just a modicum of English?" Sometimes when I answer their question with a negative, they will try to squeeze some Spanish out of me by saying, "No leetle Spanish? A leetle beet?" Then I indignantly reply while shrugging my shoulders, "Why would I know Spanish? I was born in an English speaking country." See the Appendix for an article I wrote on this subject for my pharmacy school paper, and you will see, there is a lot more to retail pharmacy than meets the eye. (Appendix D) We must be multitalented, to put it mildly. Sure we have techs helping us, but that presents a whole host of potential problems itself. Techs can very often be more of a curse than a blessing.

Advice for Pharmacy Technicians

"The ultimate result of shielding men from the effects of folly is to fill the world with fools."

- Herbert Spencer

Erik Brady and Kevin McCoy wrote an article in USA Today in February 2008 titled Drugstore Chains Rely on Pharmacy Technicians where they underlined the important role techs play in retail pharmacy. "When Americans bring prescriptions to their neighborhood pharmacies, odds are the person in the white lab coat who greets them and enters the prescription in the computer is not a pharmacist. Neither, most likely, is the person who puts the pills in the medicine vial. They're probably pharmacy technicians, in some cases teenagers with no more than high school diplomas." [1]

They quoted Paul Doering, a University of Florida pharmacy professor as stating, "The nations' state legislatures should raise standards by requiring technicians to pass a standardized certification exam." The authors also reported that, "...a USA Today review of pharmacy board records in 10 states found numerous cases in which pharmacists did not catch technician errors. In a typical example, Massachusetts's pharmacy board records show an unidentified technician 'entered the information incorrectly into the computer'

---

1   http://www.usatoday.com/money/industries/health/2008-02-12-pharma-cy-technicians_N.htm

in the prescription a CVS pharmacy dispensed to Shaun Taylor. The Kingston man suffered breathing difficulties that required hospital treatment in 2005 after he was given a Fentanyl® painkiller skin patch three times stronger than prescribed…" Stories like these are a dime a dozen.

In May 2007, "…CVS suspended pharmacy technician Katie Dudash from its Euclid, Ohio store after learning that she was involved in administering a lethal dose of medication to a child while she worked as a technician at Rainbow Babies & Children's Hospital in Cleveland. The baby, who was getting chemotherapy treatment, died three days later because of the mix-up." [2] I myself once caught a tech tripling an antibiotic suspension for an infant on my watch. Unfortunately, I have not always been so successful.

Randy Brown, the Pharmacy Technician Program Director at the MedVance Institute (a tech training school) in Houston, TX stated techs' role well, "A pharmacy technician is there to serve the pharmacist." He stipulated, "This isn't a job for everybody. It's for self-starters, people who are easily motivated. Being science and math oriented is a plus, since that's the bulk of what we deal with… you need to be able to do simple multiplication and division in your head."

For example, how many pills does John Doe need if he's taking three pills per day for 30 days? Brown says, "If that kind of math doesn't suit you, this might not be right for you." He added, "This is also a job that requires strong people skills. When you're working in retail pharmacy, you have to deal with patients all day long." He concluded by adding that most health care related jobs require working flexible hours, and that careers in pharmacy are no exception. "Hospitals and pharmacies for the most part never close, so (techs) have to be willing to give up a holiday or work late," Brown said. [3]

---

2   http://www.usatoday.com/money/industries/health/2008-02-24-emily_N.htm

3   http://www.allalliedhealthschools.com/faqs/pharmacy-technician-interview

I would argue that, for the most part, a bad tech is usually the reflection of lousy pharmacists who have trained and worked with them, or good pharmacists who are unwilling to properly train them for whatever reason. Having said that, very few of the techs that I have worked with have been competent, or even hard working, and far too many of them were simply hopeless. It is remarkable how rare it is to find a well trained one.

According to the U.S. Bureau of Labor Statistics, median hourly wages of techs in May 2008 were $13.32. The middle 50 percent earned between $10.95 and $15.88, the lowest 10 percent earned less than $9.27, and the highest 10 percent earned more than $18.98.[4] Salary.com listed the 2007 U.S. average as $27,641 with the lowest 10 percent making less than $21,663, and the highest 10 percent earning more than $34,544. Certification, evening or weekend hours, and union membership typically contribute to increased pay.

When I was a tech in the mid 90's I made around $8 per hour, and I knew my place in the pharmaceutical hierarchy. I had enough respect for the pharmacist and his knowledge, education, and experience to never think of equating myself with him. Intuitively, I knew that he was paid for what he learned during his grueling years in pharmacy school, and that I was previously a stock-boy with no knowledge of pharmacology, therapeutics, drug kinetics, etc. I was his assistant, period. My purpose was to make his job easier.

Thankfully, states are finally beginning to require that techs pass the Pharmacy Technician Certification Board (PTCB) exam. My hope in this chapter is to illustrate through anecdotes what an incompetent tech is, show what each one was missing, and thus provide guidance for those who, for whatever reason, may not realize it, thus awakening them and allowing them to make the necessary corrections for improvement.

For those of you techs who think to yourself, "Hey! I do everything that the pharmacist does except verify the finished product. Why shouldn't I make more?" Let me warn you, with all sincerity, that

4   http://www.bls.gov/oco/ocos325.htm

you really have no idea the difference between being the tech filling the script versus the person in charge who is responsible for patient safety while keeping in mind medical ethics, state law, company policy, and triple checking your work to make sure you did it right. Pharmacists have much going on in their heads. Trust me, I have spent a good deal of time in both pairs of shoes. Besides, all you have to do is get through pharmacy school and become licensed if you wish to make more money.

Pharmacists have to consider drug interactions, drug side effects, the patient's age (especially if very young or very old), ways to cut down financial costs to the patient, third party insurance issues, supervisor's orders, inventory matters, frequent corporate memos, company based learning programs (CBLs), multiple interruptions, and on and on and on. All of this must be done twelve hours per day often with no breaks depending on which company you work for. Like Dr. Grant said in Jurassic Park after giving his chilling velociraptor speech to the bratty kid, "So, you know, show a little respect, okay?"

The first thing a tech must get in their mind is the hierarchy, and their role as assistant helping to make the pharmacist's job easier. I was glad to do it, and took pride in doing it. It was my job to count quickly by fives, answer phones, and ring people up at the register, not his. Following are some basic rules I came up with for the conduct of techs.

Whenever possible, rescue the pharmacist from the register, and answer the phone ASAP. They will love you for this. Think of yourself as the first line of defense. You are responsible for promptly and politely greeting the patients as they hand you their rx. You have to make sure that it is legible. Make sure you can read their name, as well as the doctor's name, and, if not, clearly write them on the rx.

Also, ask the patient their date of birth and write that on the rx, as well as any drug allergies they may have. Ask if they have been to your pharmacy before, and if not, add them to your system. Then be sure to find out whether or not the requested drug is in stock.

A good knowledge of brand and generic drug names is useful here. Do all of this before they leave your pharmacy, and be sure to ask the patient if they wish to wait or come back later. This gives the pharmacist all of the info needed including how much time he or she has to fill the script.

The best way to do all of this is to type up the rx as you are asking these questions. This way much can be verified before they ever depart. The last thing you want is to get stuck without a pivotal piece of necessary info, or be unable to fill the rx for some reason, and then have to wait until the patient returns, in which case they will be quite upset, to say the least, because this will extend their wait time.

Once the patient leaves, you should practically be finished typing and can go right on to counting out the medication. All the pharmacist should have to do is scan the patient profile for any potential interactions, verify your work, and then bag the rx. A good tech can complete this entire process in just two or three minutes. They should be able to move quickly, accurately, and multitask.

If you cannot multitask, then don't even apply for the job. This ability is crucial. There is no reason while on hold with an insurance company, which will be often, that you cannot also type, run the register, or answer the other phones. I cannot tell you how many times I have had two phones attached to my head while typing at the same time. I must have looked like a pharmanut.

Of course, when it's busy, then it is a bit of a different story. Simply take the rxs one by one while writing the aforementioned necessary info on them, and hand them off to the pharmacist while he or she types. Do not forget to indicate which rxs are waiters (they will be back shortly), and which will be picked up later in the day.

Once the train of drop-offs is gone, then either begin counting pills, or rescue the pharmacist from typing, whatever their preference. Part of the job description of a tech is learning multiple ways to do the same thing because you must cater to the pharmacist you are working with at the time. As each rx is verified, then grab the ones that the patients are waiting for and begin ringing them up.

If someone has a question for the pharmacist, then just tell the person that the pharmacist will be with him or her as soon as possible. Do not shout from across the pharmacy, "This customer has a question for you!" Just let the pharmacist know as soon, and as calmly as you can; remember, they're concentrating.

Few things are more irritating than to be talking to someone on the phone, and your tech is asking you a question at the same time. "Can you not see my mouth moving and hear the words coming out, and this phone attached to my head?!" Unbelievably, I have even had fellow pharmacists do this to me. Interruptions are the number one cause of QREs.

During the chaos, the pharmacist may get stuck ringing people up at the register. If you notice this, then drop what you are doing, unless in the middle of counting pills, and rescue him or her, otherwise the assembly line gets clogged. The pharmacist has to be free to verify rxs if things are going to run smoothly. The reason we do not want you to stop counting is because you may either make a mistake by miscounting, or because it is unwise to leave an unlabeled bottle with pills in it. QREs make pharmacists extremely cranky.

I am a big believer in 'Get it done.' Some techs have their duties down to a science and thus they pace themselves so as to wrap up whatever task they are working on just in time for lunch break, or the end of their shift. Do not drag your feet. Work fast, get everything done ASAP, and then relax once you are caught up.

There is also a standard rule I enforce when filling a suspension rx that requires purified water be added to it. Do not add the water until you see the whites of the patient's eyes. This is because once the water is added the clock starts ticking. Sure most antibiotic suspensions do not even require refrigeration and can stay at room temperature for several days, but what if the patient's parents never come to pick it up? Then you have to hope that you become fortunate enough to get yet another rx for the same exact drug and quantity in about 10 to 14 days, otherwise you have to trash it and that is a sad waste.

The National Pharmacy Technician Association (NPTA) and the US Department of Labor reported more than 39,000 pharmacy tech job openings since 2006, and they expect the field to grow 27% or more through 2014. We can ill afford to continue down this path of low expectations and ineptitude. On May 7, 2007 Mike Johnson, CPhT wrote an article in Drug Topics Magazine entitled "It's Time to Standardize Pharmacy Technician Training", in which he referenced an ABC News report on medication errors caused by pharmacy professionals that ran on March 30, 2007. "The network ran three separate investigative reports- on Good Morning America, World News Tonight, and 20/20- all on the same day, presenting a damaging portrayal of pharmacy practice." [5]

For this reason, among others, The NPTA took the position that individuals should be required to complete a standardized education/ training program, pass a validated competency-based exam, and be registered with their state pharmacy board in order to practice as pharmacy technicians." Here! Here! Mike, who is chairman and CEO of the NPTA, concluded by saying, "Pharmacy techs are a critical part of the pharmacy team and for them to be efficient and effective team members, standardized education is necessary."

Now to be fair, a good pharmacist will help the tech. If the tech is getting slammed, then the pharmacist should not only type, but also not be afraid to run the cash register as well. I have actually had floater pharmacists (think substitute teacher) proclaim to my face that they positively refuse to run the register, as if it is so beneath them that they would rather die than suffer such injustice. This is pathetic.

Another problem that seems to be rampant in the retail pharmacy world is the basic ability to alphabetize. I have had so much trouble

---

5   http://drugtopics.modernmedicine.com/drugtopics/Miscellaneous/Its-time-to-standardize-tech-training/ArticleStandard/Article/detail/423925

with this simple requirement in my experiences that I have seriously contemplated, after having tried everything else, posting the standard elementary school wall decorative of the entire alphabet with large case letters adjacent to small case letters for quick and easy reference for those who seem to need extra help. It is irksome, to say the least, when fundamental things are not done like alphabetization, proper numerization, cleaning, typing, stocking supplies, answering the phone in a timely fashion, etc. Basic expectations not met, because they are basic, are difficult to tolerate.

Talking to patients on the phone is a basic tech duty as well. Most retail pharmacy companies require the staff to call patients at home after failing to pick up their rx after one week. We have to ask them if they intend to pick it up, or not. If they say they will be in to get it, then we will hold it for a few more days. If they say they will not need it, then we reverse the claim in the computer, and then place the drug back on the shelf. After ten days, we put it back regardless; otherwise we run the risk of insurance fraud.

Counting accurately on a consistent basis is also a problem for some people. I had a tech that regularly miscounted even controlled drugs far too often. She would get really offended and positively angry with me for double-checking her work including the counting of controlled drugs, and yet would continue to foul up. Good pharmacists will always double-count controlled medications. Even if this tech had been accurate, she still would not have been justified in her indignance, but she often actually did miscount the controlled drugs. She couldn't even get the child proof versus easy open caps correct on a consistent basis!

After bringing these errors to her attention she would often throw a fit. Thin-skinned people seldom improve because their attitude prohibits an honest self-assessment. What I never was sure of was whether she was angry with herself for continually screwing up such a simple duties, or if she was mad at me for having the audacity to verify her accuracy and correct her. Being that she was not very accurate, I would hope it was the former, but I am fairly certain it was the later.

After one of her tantrums, I told her about an Ohio pharmacist who was sentenced to jail in 2009 for involuntary manslaughter of a two year old child. [6] He received 6 years in jail, along with 6 years probation, plus thousands of dollars in fines as well as community service because his tech screwed up a compounded rx. News stories on rx errors caused by techs are voluminous.

This is not to say that pharmacists do not also make errors themselves. All I am pointing out here is that our techs mistakes are also our mistakes. It is we who are held responsible when something goes wrong, and here I had a delicate tech whose ego could not handle my checking of her work. Clearly she was in the wrong business. Retail pharmacy is a field where constant scrutiny, evaluation, and constructive criticism are ingrained.

Another basic expectation that every tech must master is the typing of the directions (i.e., sig) on the rx into the computer, which will eventually be printed on the label and attached to the patient's drug vial. The sig nomenclature must be mastered by all techs. This exposes yet another area lacking among far too many techs, and that is proper spelling and grammar. Would you want to take pills from someone who typed on your vial, "take dialy?" If they are careless about that, then what else are they careless about?

Reliability is also huge, and is especially more so than in any other medical branch. Pharmacists need the techs to show up on time, stay until they are scheduled to stay, and not call in sick more frequently than a sorority applicant during pledge week. A pharmacy simply cannot operate efficiently without the techs being there to help prevent the pharmacist from getting bogged down in trivial things that prevent rxs from being filled in a timely manner.

---

6   http://blog.cleveland.com/metro/2009/05/expharmacist_eric_cropp_found.html

I have had techs actually alter their schedule behind my back without telling me, and then not show up for work at all. They would automatically give themselves days off on holidays without even asking me first. I had others who would call in sick whenever their dog was sick!

These are the archetypal long-term techs who have been in a certain pharmacy so long that they feel they are the manager, and you are just the latest pharmacist to come along. They know they will be there long after you're gone, and they'll be damned if they're going to listen to anything you have to say. In these battles, so far, I have won. I displaced two prima donnas from the same pharmacy once. It was a brutal battle, both times, but getting them out of there was worth it. Don't fuss with the pharmacist is a tough lesson to have to teach, but a necessary one at times.

Then you have the techs that wish to challenge you and your knowledge. This is often a sucker punch, and so they may get you the first time. I then incorporate the advice of Mark Twain, who said, "If you suspect that someone has taken a shot at you, then wait for the opportunity and hit them with a ton of bricks." Any tech that has tried to expose me for an incompetent, has quickly realized their own profound lack of ability and knowledge because I poignantly underline it for them at every single opportunity, which turns out to be much more frequent than they would have cared to realize.

Techs, no matter how knowledgeable you may think you are, and no matter how dumb you think your pharmacist is, trust me, you don't know what they know. It may be tough at times, but unless they're a *pharmanazi* who treats you poorly, then show them the proper respect. Some pharmacists' skin are thicker than others, but eventually we all get sick of techs challenging our authority, and questioning our expertise on a daily basis. What follows is a conversation between *the* prima donna tech (now a felon) who felt I had trespassed into her pharmacy, and almost daily tried to display her acumen by challenging me. All she showed was her lack of it, and one day I had had enough.

Patient: "What does grapefruit juice do to my drugs that I can't drink it?"

Me: "It affects the enzymes in your body that break down the drug thus making it work either too well or not well enough."

Tech: "Not to disagree with you, but isn't it that grapefruit juice affects the drug itself?"

Me: "Well, how do drugs come to work in the body? Through chemical reactions that break it down thus making it work biologically. Ever take basic chemistry? What is it that provides the impetus for a chemical reaction to take place? Right, enzymes. The grapefruit juice does one of two things in regard to the enzymes, which remember now, facilitate chemical reactions causing the drug to work. The first is called enzyme induction, which, to make a long story short, causes the drug to work not as well as it would otherwise. The opposite reaction is called enzyme inhibition, and does what? Right, causes the drug to work too well, more or less."

Befuddled Tech: "…….."

Of course, all of this is bland detail, and moot if the underlying concept is not understood. A tech's purpose is to aid the pharmacist and make their job easier, personality conflicts not withstanding. As with most jobs, tasks must be completed quickly and accurately, you must be reliable and dependable (this is especially important in any branch of medicine), you should be courteous and polite to patients, you should respect the pharmacist's position at the least and the person at best, and you certainly should never place blame on anyone in the pharmacy for anything that goes wrong; save that for their counseling session.

A pharmacy is a very small work environment, and the interactions between the employees are intimate. It is dreadful for people who do not get along, and dislike one another, to work in a pharmacy together. This is the only branch of the medical world set in a retail environment. There are unique dynamics at place-interpersonal, professional, and otherwise. Different sets of rules apply. Remember, one of the challenges of being a tech is learning several different methods to accomplish basically the same thing because every pharmacist has the right to require certain things be done his or her own way, for the most part, and it is your duty to cater to whomever it is you are working with at the time.

Some signs of a lazy tech:

- Goes to the restroom 15 minutes before their shift is over and comes back just in time to punch out.

- Acts like they did not know how to do something, to have forgotten how to do it, or claims that the policy must have recently changed.

- Blames everyone but themselves for mishaps.

- Frequently calls in sick for frivolous reasons, such as their pet being sick.

- Pretends to be unaware of something such as not noticing a customer waiting at the window.

- Consistently gives a much longer wait time than you do (sometimes double) at the drop off window.

- Makes excuse after excuse: "I would do it if only I had the time," "No one ever showed me that before," "I thought we weren't allowed to do that," "I'm still getting used to the system," "You make me nervous," blah, blah, blah. My buddy Ben Franklin said, "He who is good at making excuses is seldom good at anything else."

- Looks at you when the phone rings to see if you are going to go for it first.

Following are just a handful of basic guidelines from a handout I made once for my staff of BASIC tech duties. For the complete list see the Appendix (Appendix E).

- Acknowledge person at the counter as soon as they walk up (if busy say, "I'll be right there" or "I'll be right with you", etc.).

- At pick up, always make sure you have the correct patient vis-à-vis their date of birth, address, etc.,

- When putting the order away, always place new drugs behind the old ones on the shelf, and always place in alphabetical order.

- We should never run out of supplies, especially during season.

Anyone who can master the complete list has a shot at being a pretty good tech, but that is only according to me. What about a more universal system? Well, in February 2008, in response to the death of a two year-old from a tech error in Rep. LaTourette's (R-OH) district, the Congressman introduced the Pharmacy Technician Training and Registration Act of 2008 (HR 5491). [7]

The legislation created a grant program for states to establish tech registration programs. In exchange for the federal grant money, states need to require certification and training of techs as well as adverse event reporting of tech errors. Trust me, many of us in the field were shouting, "Eureka!"

---

7   http://www.opencongress.org/bill/110-h5491/show

"20 Years" Experience

"There are three things extremely hard: steel, a diamond, and to know one's self."

- Benjamin Franklin

Every time a tech has boasted to me about having "20 years" experience, I have been gravely disappointed. If no one had told me beforehand, and all I had to go on was my own observations, then I would have guessed that they had no more than two weeks experience under their belts. If a tech brags to you about having "20 years" experience, then just assume that they need to be retrained, and prepare to do everything yourself. If running is an option, I recommend that also.

Sadly, most pharmacists are either too lazy or apathetic to properly train their staff. I worked overtime once with a tech who had been at that pharmacy for a full year. She did not know how to put paper in the printer. I repeat, she did not know how to put paper in the printer! This is that particular pharmacist's fault; however, as Benjamin Franklin once stated, "There are lazy minds as well as lazy bodies," and she could have learned most of the basics on her own. These seasoned "20-year" techs are a prime example of this in the retail pharmacy world.

In my experience, "20 year" techs can barely input a new rx without getting stumped about half a dozen times during the process. Shouldn't a tech with this much experience know how to add allergies to a patient's profile? Shouldn't they know the sig for 'allergy'? Should they know that you need the Dr.'s DEA number in order to get a rx to go through the patient's insurance, and should you have to tell them to call the doctor's office to get it? How about the ability to check drug prices? Oh, and when you tell them to take out the trash you had better mention emptying the shredder too. Yes, you have to tell them to do that otherwise confetti overflow is the result, and your pharmacy will look like the day after Mardi Gras.

I have personally trained techs from scratch who, after two or three months, were better than these pinheads. It took my latest tech of "20 years" experience a full ten months of training to finally figure out how to put staples in the damn stapler! I wish I was making this stuff up. Clearly, she was not only cerebrally challenged, but also stunningly lazy.

These bastions of limitless experience are also very often extremely slow for some reason. They move like a tortoise with three broken legs. Sometimes I feel like I'm in a George Romero movie, Pharmacy of the Dead, or something. In fact, you could say that if they moved any slower they would actually be un-filling rxs. Often they take a good 5 to 10 minutes to type in a simple Z-Pac® rx as they stand there with a befuddled look on their face as if they're trying to work the controls on the Millennium Falcon for the first time, all the while furrowing their brows in a vain attempt to understand and overcome various obstacles they encounter along the way. Sadly, some old-timer pharmacists I've seen are just as bad.

It is truly lamentable how few "20 year" tech veterans have an adequate knowledge of the proper sig jargon. It is even more remarkable how few can type a complete sentence without spelling or grammatical errors. I had one ask me what ">" meant. She also had to ask me the difference between PM (evening) and HS (bedtime). I am not kidding.

"Twenty years" experience and they have to ask me such things as, "What does BID (twice daily) mean?" "How many is 'one tablet three times daily for ten days'?" "How many milliliters is one tablespoon?" "How many days supply is a Medrol® dosepak?" or a "Z-Pac®?" Once I was asked, "What is 7 times 6?" These are all things that ought to be completely mastered with no more than three months experience. My twelve-year-old toddler could have answered the last one…five years ago!

I have worked for companies that allow me to assist busier stores with functions such as data entry and verification of rxs, and I would have to say that close to 50% of them require some type of correction. Anyone know who Officer Barbrady from South Park is? How about Chief Wiggum from the Simpsons? If not, then think of us pharmacists as Clark W. Griswald, and we have to work with cousin Eddy all day long.

These are the sort of techs who mispronounce drugs like, "Lisnopril," "Citralpram," "Simvastin," "Pravastin," etc. When they say "acrost" or "pacific" in the place of across and specific, then you know you have a real thoroughbred. Many techs I have worked with are mumbly, shy, can barely communicate, and thus hate calling patients. I can just see them huddled with their buddies at the mall grunting at one another like the "Fierce People" from The Emerald Forest in some sort of Mallrats II- The Quest for Fire scene.

While bragging about her "20 years" experience, one tech struggled to type a simple rx into the computer. Again, it was a simple Z-Pac®. As if that wasn't bad enough, she also had a contrarian attitude, as if she were in charge. She would even tell me not to order certain drugs, because she was concerned about our inventory getting out of control. We had just opened. One-third of our shelves were empty. We had no stinking inventory.

Other times she barked that we needed to order certain drugs; just an insolent PITA (Pain In The Ass) to be sure. Few things are as irksome as a know-it-all who knows almost nothing at all. At this point, if anyone brags to me about "20 years" experience, I'm just going to prescribe myself high velocity intracranial lead therapy.

"What does AD mean?" was the favorite question from my tech of "20 years" experience. "Um, 'As Directed,'" is all my disgust will allow me to muster for an answer. It could also mean right ear, but only if you're filling a rx for eardrops. She must have asked me that question about half a dozen times in the course of a year. Astonished, yet? Wait, it gets better.

One time we ran out of rx bags. We literally could not bag the rxs, so I asked her why this was the case and her unbelievable response was, "Well, I didn't know we were getting low." I kept my composure, but in my brain I was screaming, "HELLO! HELLO!!! That's your job you colossal dope! You vapid useless pile of bone and skin!" You have to understand, imagine being stuck in a tiny little room having to work all day every day with the buffoonery of Forest Gump suffering from a concussion.

After "20 years," a tech ought to know almost as much as a pharmacist as far as the basics go such as how to check in a drug order, how to send back expired drugs, how to deal with insurance problems, how to fix printer malfunctions, how to handle drug recalls, etc. Even a knowledge of the most common drugs can occur if one is only minimally observant with a mere hint of curiosity and interest in their job. In all honesty, the main problem with this particular person was her remarkable laziness, and she probably feigned some of her astonishing ignorance for a lack of desire to work.

If you were just a pharmacy cashier or clerk before you came to the pharmacy, then fine, but don't brag to me all the time about your vast knowledge and experience. It also shows a lack of desire to learn, or thinking that it is not something that needs to be known. One of the favorite excuses for not knowing how to do the simplest things is, "Well, I never learned that because of all of my other responsibilities." That excuse had been used so often by one tech that I began to wonder what these phantom responsibilities were. Judging from her abilities, I would say they were mostly cash register oriented. She was upper-middle aged, but moved like she was 110.

It's one thing to be slow; it's another to be inert. A slug in a salt mine could move faster.

She was another one who thought it easier to ask rather than investigate herself. With that ever so familiar vacuous look on her face she would blurt out questions about something without any basis for a reference whatsoever.

"What happened to this?" she would yell from across the pharmacy.

"What are you referring to, exactly?" I'd inquire.

"This Carafate® suspension," she'd reply.

"Okay....what about it?"

"What happened to it?"

My pre-migraine aura would begin to kick in, "Um, I have no idea, what do you think happened to it?"

"It's gone now," she bluntly states as if it's in the ether somewhere.

"But aren't you currently holding it in your hand?" I asked.

"Well, I was going to fill it. We ordered it for a patient and it came in today, but now it's not in the computer," she helplessly stated.

"Ahhh...well, see I haven't been here since Thursday, that was four days ago. I have no idea what you're talking about. Let's see what happ....oh look! There it is! It's in the *fill* queue!"

She then muttered, "Oh, it must have automatically gone in there after I checked in the drug order, you think? Does the computer do that automatically?"

The migraine is at full force by now, "You're asking me? I've been here six months; you've been here '20 years'. Yes, it automatically goes into *fill* after you check in the order." I am ready to cry from the pain at this point.

When I started with this particular company, the pharmacy supervisor (think Zap Branigan) told me she was an "ace tech" with tons of experience and knowledge. Come to think of it, he would have made one hell of a car salesman, or better yet, a talent scout for the Detroit Lions. After hassling him for a full year, and explaining that she was a "cancer on the pharmacy," he finally transferred her to another store where she thoroughly tortured the staff there. Last I heard, they had her solely working the cash register, and she had done that so well that she was written up for gross incompetence after dispensing the wrong rx bags to the wrong people.

As expected, the pharmacists there cursed the supervisor for dropping her at their doorstep. In fact, one of them said to me, "She should have been fired a long time ago." Yes, exactly, but why wasn't she? How do these boobs persist in this branch of medicine?

If the populace knew what was going on here regarding incompetent techs, there would be riots in the streets. Then again, my former supervisor should have been fired as well. Why, you ask? Well, the cronyism was vile, but perhaps not worthy of dismissal. Maybe gross incompetence since he either made things worse by transferring bad apples from store to store, or refrained from doing hardly anything at all including reading or responding to desperate phone calls and emails pleading for help.

Periodically, my former useless tech with vast skills acquired over "20 years" would visit me asking about our volume wondering if we were busy enough to transfer her back. Sure, over my dead body. I would rather piss broken glass than to work with her again. To this day she almost certainly has no idea that it was I who facilitated her removal. The supervisor gave her the impression that she was no longer needed at my store because of the low volume, and that her services were required elsewhere. If she had a clue that it was I who started that ball rolling, then she would not have wasted her time trying to slither her way back.

At that time I honestly would have preferred to leave the company and quit rather than deal with her again. Come to think of it, thank God I no longer work under the supervision of Zap. His repeated poor judgments aged me horribly during the time I suffered there.

All too often, a burnt out office cashier is transferred to the pharmacy thinking it will be a good place to relax and take it easy. They bring with them a lassie faire attitude not realizing the immense responsibility that comes with now being an active member the medical community. They also come with disgruntled baggage that one attains only after many grueling years at a customer service counter.

When they say that they have "20 years" tech experience, what they probably mean is that they have worked for that same company for that period of time. They are also trying to somehow prevent you from noticing their incompetence. It stems from an inferiority complex of some kind. What they fail to realize is that they cause the opposite to happen; they highlight their lack of skill and knowledge because of the expectations that claim brings. When you cannot work the friggin' stapler, or whole puncher after two decades, well then you need to find a new line of work. Based on what I witnessed with this person, I would recommend paint-drying observer; either that, or retire.

Another possible factor is that the training they received for those "20 years" was poor and practically non-existent. Maybe the particular pharmacists tutoring them were horrible trainers, or, after some time, they mistakenly figured it would be easier to just do everything themselves, and allow the tech to live the delusion that they are competent. Perhaps futility just eventually set in.

There is a universal law that these pharmacists are forgetting, and that is that low expectations breed incompetence. This is why all of the techs I have trained from scratch have razzled and dazzled anytime they've rendered their services elsewhere. I do not meant to toot my own horn, but the results speak for themselves.

Sure, training techs is a pain, but not training them is even more of a hassle, especially when it gets busy during season. The last thing you want when it's crunch time in your pharmacy is to have an undependable tech who does little more than just get in your way, makes a plethora of mistakes, constantly interrupts you with dumb questions from across the room, slows down your progress, blames everyone else for their shortcomings, and in effect actually makes your job harder. To hear them tell it, they are perfect human beings who never make mistakes. I cannot tell you how many times I have heard, "It wasn't me! I didn't do that! I never do that. It was so and so's fault."

If you think that tech trainers are the solution, then let me say this, I have yet to see one that could live up to the name. If you are very fortunate, then your tech will evaluate them self, especially after observing someone competent, and come to the realization that they need to get their act together. Sadly, this seldom ever occurs.

Most techs are not academics, and did not get into pharmacy because of their desire to join a branch of medicine. More likely they thought it would be an easy job. This explains the incessant inquiries by the work release deli guys wanting to know if there is an opening. A smart company policy would be to mandate that all techs periodically work in different pharmacies to broaden their horizons (i.e., see how it's done). Thank goodness states are beginning to require rx tech registration, and hopefully soon certification.

However, at the end of the day, if they can get away with less, then they will. Many have absolutely no incentive to improve because they consider the discrepancy between their salary and yours an injustice, and figure you ought to work a lot harder than they do anyway. Some things you can do is cut their hours, give them less desirable shifts, share them with the grocery department, and basically wean them out of your pharmacy.

After "20 years" too many still do not realize that we are paid for our knowledge, and that a natural hierarchy exists in the retail pharmacy world. Not to mention most pharmacists borrowed heavily to get through school and are now burdened with at least $100,000 in debt. Were they to risk such a position for their education and career, then perhaps they could better relate and even sympathize with us.

Those techs who have been in the same pharmacy for a long period of time are the worst not just because they are set in their ways, but because they think that their seniority gives them a voice comparable and perhaps even superior to yours within that particular company. Do not bend to them because they will take it and run; all you'll see is a roadrunner dust cloud.

A pharmacist with one-minute experience has seniority over a tech with 30 years experience, period. Establish your superiority as soon as you see a hint of their conceit. They must understand that your word is final; there is no argument, there is no debate, and if they disregard your instructions and do what they want to do, then write them up and explain that this is intolerable and unacceptable. Three strikes and you're out.

If the desire is there, but they simply lack the ability to learn, then the same rules apply. Either way it is our responsibility to do what is best for the pharmacy and the customers. I once wrote a letter to the Vice President and CEO of the Florida Pharmacy Association after a particularly bad day with Mrs. Twenty Years Experience pleading for some form of standards to be passed by the state legislators vis-à-vis techs. My letter and his response can be found in the appendix (Appendix F).

Pharmacy Technician Anecdotes

"A wise man knows that he knows not..."

- Aristotle

My first uncomfortable experience with a tech was one who not only was the spitting image of Roseanne Barr, but also had her same attitude when she played a waitress on her TV show. I would print out months' worth of hourly break downs of rx filling, and show her the typical busy and slow times. I then asked her if she wouldn't mind taking her break during the slow time. While walking away from me, she defiantly murmured, "No."

In her mind I was "the boss man" commanding her what to do, including when she was permitted to go on break no less! What a lot of techs do not realize is that it is not what is best for them; it is what is best for the pharmacy that matters. It is the duty of the pharmacy manager to keep the pharmacy functioning as efficiently as possible.

What she failed to understand was that this was no power trip I was on, it was a rational request based on concrete business trends, and that this was what was best for the pharmacy and the patients. Schedules can change at any time, and a tech must be available for any shift. This is something expected of all techs everywhere. Why should I be working alone during what was accurately predicted to be a busy time, thus causing customers to have to wait longer to get their rxs, and increasing the likelihood of a QRE? Conversely, why should she work during a predictably slow hour?

She was also horrible with the personal calls. Like clock work, every day around 5:00 to 5:30 PM (the busiest time of the day), her husband or one of her kids would call just to say hello, or ask what was for dinner. This despite the fact that she was about to get off at 6:00 PM! She made many personal calls herself as well. I will never forget how, at a very busy moment, she actually had two phones to her ears at the same time, and both were personal calls.

Phone ringing is a major distraction. Sure, it is a part of the job, but all the more reason not to make it worse. This tech augmented it. Distractions lead to QREs for techs as well as pharmacists. This is especially unnerving if you are not a phone person, and the ringing of a phone sends an impulse down your spine that twists it into a pretzel.

Her boorishness and insubordinate attitude often caused her to lash out at the patients. I wanted to speak up, but hesitated because she was a close personal friend of my partner who was the pharmacy manager at the time. A piece of advice for pharmacists, never hire a personal friend to work with you in the pharmacy. Not only will it make everyone else working back there uncomfortable, but it will backfire on you too.

Pharmacy is a field where constructive criticism is part of the job. A friend, not familiar with this concept and not educated at a pharmacy school, may not respond very well to this. Everyone behind a pharmacy counter has to be closely monitored, their work closely scrutinized, and their performance constantly critiqued. This is hard to do with a close friend, especially if they are poor at their job.

I transferred out of that pharmacy after one year of putting up with her. My next tech was the worst I have ever seen in all of my years in retail pharmacy. I lasted there about two months and, in fact, ended up leaving the company at that point.

Honest to God, this tech was utterly useless, and even more stunningly lazy than Mrs. Twenty Years. Stephen King could not have written a more horrifying character. One day, I swear, she spent more time on her cell phone with personal calls, than she did off of the phone. Often she would leave the pharmacy for about thirty minutes at a time unannounced, and even delivered the pharmacy manager's paycheck to her house while on the clock. Rumor had it they were lovers, but here we go again with personal hiring. She would then go on break after returning.

One time the printer beeped that it was empty, and I, being new there, asked her where the printer paper was. She went on another thirty-minute magical mystery tour, and came back with a single pack of paper, and then slammed it on the counter. Surely she knew the printer was still empty, hence the previous beeping and impetus of my question, but she did not fill the printer. She was, in affect, saying to me, "You do it."

Again, I would have been tougher on her, but not only was she close to my partner on a personal level, but she also had everyone's pity due to her ailing parents. Apparently, they were on the verge of death. I had worked overtime at that store a year before, and heard the same story. Her folks had been on their deathbed, by that time, for well over a year at the very least. I had never before, and have never since, seen any worker, pharmacy related or not, as lazy, pathetic, and useless. I still shudder when I think about what it was like to work with her, and would rather chew broken glass than ever do so again.

So, then I transfer over to another company that assures me that I am getting their best store vis-à-vis the outstanding techs. Little did I know that I was being dropped into the lion's den. This would become a trend from company to company.

One tech ended up filing charges with the company claiming that I created "an uncomfortable work environment." I used bad words that offended his delicate sensibilities. Sadly, we pharmacists are a profane bunch at times. Working retail long enough will cause even the most sainted to drop a swear word periodically.

We had to sit with a couple of higher-ups, and the result was that he now carried a tape recorder with him at all times. I cannot tell you how many times he bungled it around, and dropped it on the floor blowing his cover. Yeah, not exactly 007. There are three fictional characters that I think of immediately when I think of him: Otis vis-à-vis Ned Beatty in Superman, with the laziness and stupidity of a real life version of Homer Simpson, along with the vileness of Newman from the Seinfeld show.

He ended up transferring thinking that he was leaving me high and dry; all the while I provoked the move from behind the scenes. I heard that he not only filled charges against the company for transferring him "involuntarily" (he unwittingly went to an extremely busy store), but also was trying to claim workman's comp for hurting his back. Last I heard he "accidentally" hurt himself yet again on the job, and is now on disability. I imagine he will remain as productive as he ever was when I had the unpleasant privilege of working with him. In response to the profanity charge I quote Mark Twain, "Under certain circumstances…profanity provides a relief denied even to prayer."

The other tech was the prima donna with 10 years experience. She was seemingly much more competent, but only because he had her morning routine memorized to a tee. This initially gave the impression that she was an ace tech. She also presented herself very professionally. It took time to notice her deficiency in having to improvise on the spot. Anything not memorized beforehand paralyzed her. To put an indelicate point on it, she could not think, or to say it more kindly, could not problem solve. She was the sort of tech who had been at the same store so long that she felt it was her pharmacy and that she ran the show. In fact, those were her exact words.

After 007 had been ousted, she made a comment to someone (who later testified against her in a company investigation) that she was upset and said, "I lost a tech because of him." What does it say when a tech laments that they "lost a tech"? It sounded like she felt that not only was the pharmacy hers, but so was the staff! This was when the QRE's really began to fly. All of a sudden, and only on my shifts, she was making several catastrophic mistakes multiple times per day. It was intentional. I am convinced of that fact, and still have evidence to this day that proves it; evidence that my superiors at the time had absolutely no interest in seeing.

After tripling the dose of an infant's antibiotic suspension, I wrote her up. I had warned her many, many times before. In fact, I had pulled her aside the week before to ask if everything was okay in her life. She had serious marital problems, and was taking a lot of prescription drugs in an effort to cope. Despite pointing out each and every error, big and small, she was blasé about them. After the write up, she exploded with self-righteous indignation. "You can't write me up! I haven't been written up in 10 years!" I explained to her that I was not trying to make history, and that her ego was not a concern to me. She stormed out of the pharmacy with rx in hand, which is illegal by the way.

My supervisor, who was a study in duplicity, tried smoothing things over. He told me things, which I imagine he said to her as well, simply exchanging names. I know this because she went around the store bragging that I was going to be written up and disciplined by the company. Funny, that's what I heard about her. Unbelievably, it never occurred to her that someone might repeat this to me.

After two witnesses testified during a company investigation, which I had to push hard for, she was written up...several times, supposedly. Remember, my supervisor at the time was a two-faced S.O.B. Some of the things they quoted her as saying included, "I run that pharmacy", "I'm going to get his ass for this", etc. Only after the other techs and grocery personnel testified on my behalf, were they forced to do something about her. The pharmacy supervisor eventually transferred her out of my pharmacy.

In the summer of 2008, she and her boyfriend were both locked up for scamming several local pharmacies out of hundreds of oxycodone pills with fake rxs.[8] Investigators said she tipped pill buyers by telling them which stores they would have the best chance of getting the fraudulent rxs filled. You see, soon after I got her expelled from my pharmacy, the supervisor unbelievably *promoted* her to tech trainer. This provided her the perfect avenue with which to scout various pharmacies ripe for the plucking.

I admit to a massive dose of schadenfreude when I heard the news of her arrest. I even went so far as to rub it into my former supervisor and district manager, both of whom paid scant attention to my complaints about her as a "bad apple." Her replacement, who testified for me and whom I had high hopes for, was a huge bust.

This tech had some serious emotional and mental problems, which ostensibly prevented her from ever coming to work on time, ever. She was late on a daily basis, that's a daily basis, sometimes by as much as two hours, and always with an elaborate excuse. At one point, I began scheduling her an hour earlier than I actually needed her. Despite that, she would still be late! She was also a very slow learner. Eventually, I had to evaluate her, and told her that her unreliability and inability to learn were troubling me. After her 90-day evaluation something amazing happened. All of these acts of God ceased and she began coming in 15 minutes early every day! My points that staying late does not make up for arriving late, and you can get your ass to work on time despite your obsessive compulsive disorder if you put your mind to it, must have resonated.

We really had to be careful because the Disabilities Act makes it impossible to fire an incompetent person if their disability is the cause for their incompetence. Nice, eh? Not long after the evaluation, all of a sudden, while still in her early 40's, she had to have a hysterectomy, and ended up being out for about a millennia. By the time she was ready to return, I had quit and begun working for yet another company. I was told that on her first day back, she did not show. They let her go the following day.

8   Liz Freeman. Naples Daily News. June 9, 2008.

Once I began working for the next company, I was relieved to not only get away from the Bizarro World I was in, but because I heard that my new tech was roundly regarded as a well-trained, super tech. You would think by now that the alarm bells should have rung in my head. Of course, she was a nightmare. This was the ever-infamous "20 years experience" tech. Yes, it has been a long haul for me.

Anyway, you have to be tough at times. Too many pharmacists have weak managerial skills, and do not do what is needed to provide what is best for the pharmacy. The tech, the store manager, and even your own feelings are secondary. As a pharmacy manager, you have to be willing and able to do what is necessary for your pharmacy and your patients. Disaster results when the heart tries to do the brain's job.

Advice for Doctors

"Doctors are men who prescribe medicines of which they know little, to cure disease of which they know less, in human beings of whom they know nothing."

- Voltaire

You need not to have worked a single day in any field of medicine to guess what the primary complaint pharmacists have in regard to medical doctors. Thanks to countless political cartoons, most laymen realize that it is the indecipherable handwriting on rxs that causes hirsutism in pharmacists. As if trying to make sense out of what often looks like a long dead alien dialect from the deepest regions of the universe is not bad enough, then we have to burn an immense amount of time calling the doctor's office, getting through to a live person, preferably one who knows what they are doing, and then getting a translation of the doodle before us.

Eventually, we may be fortunate enough to get a chance to speak to the wiz behind the curtain. Most pharmacists get the, kneel before Zod treatment from physicians; however, despite this, I still have a lot of respect for medical doctors. They are mostly exceptional people doing an extremely difficult job, and doing it, more often than not, very well. They too are overworked, especially these days. Voltaire once said, "Medicine consists of amusing the patient while nature cures the disease." I give doctors the benefit of the doubt.

An illegible rx not only causes frustration for the pharmacist who cannot read it and the patient who has to wait for the doctor's office to decode it, but it is downright hazardous and potentially lethal. A federal law needs to be passed compelling doctors to either write clearly, or type out all rxs. Currently, only a few states have such laws. Every medical school should at least offer an elective course on penmanship as part of their curriculum. Currently, only one medical school offers such a class. Consequences for prescribing with careless caveman-like handwriting need to be raised a tad.

Often, I find myself like Indiana Jones pulling the rubber band off of his little decoder book, piercing at the Egyptian hieroglyphics with sweat pouring off of his brow, tensely holding a pencil between his teeth, and trying to decipher the meaning of what lies before him. The feeling of jubilation that overcomes me when I successfully decode a rx is hard to describe in words. Just observe the look on Indy's face when the intense beam of celestial light points the way to the Lost Ark in the map room, or imagine how Howard Carter felt in 1922 when he discovered Tut's tomb. We pharmacists feel the same way after performing the Nicholas Cage-National Treasure routine in solving the M.D.'s penmanship puzzle. As you can see by my absurd and overt referencing, it can be quite exhilarating.

No one has more appreciation for the knowledge held by and hard work performed by doctors than I. Having said that, it is irksome to say the least when, in an honest attempt to get the rx right so as to not kill the patient, they act very rudely in response to my inquiries, ostensibly because of this unjustified intrusion on their time. Too many of them have a god complex, and act as though it is beneath them to speak verbally to me.

One of my proudest moments was when I put a notorious doctor in his place. For years he refused to make prior authorization (PA) calls for his own patients. This is when the insurance company wants the pharmacy to inform the doctor to call them in order to verbally authorize the rx that was written. After repeated failures by other members of the staff to get him to do this for his own patient, I took up the challenge. The conversation went like this:

JM: "Yes doctor, I have a prior authorization call for your patient."

M.D.: "What the hell are you bothering me for? Can't you call them!?"

JM: "The insurance company wants to hear from you."

M.D.: "I just asked you a yes or no question."

JM: "Well by implication the answer is obviously no."

M.D.: "You are a rude son of a bitch!"

JM: "As are you."

M.D.: "Let me talk to my patient."

After a useless five-minute conversation we were back to square one.

M.D.: "The patient ought to be able to call them himself."

JM: "But the insurance company doesn't want to speak to the patient, they want to hear from you."

M.D.: "This is ridiculous!"

JM: "Doctor, can you not make a simple phone call and authorize this medication for your own patient?"

Eventually he made the call, and within minutes he actually made a courtesy call back to our pharmacy to inform us it had been done. We were stunned, and victory was mine! I had to verbally arm wrestle with him for a while, but the mission was accomplished. I was showered with praise for days, and the staff, which was accustomed to this PITA, recounted the tale to others for weeks.

Apparently, far too many physicians feel above directly communicating with their own patients as well because I am continually baffled by the number of customers who say they have no idea what the rx is for, and do not know how to take or use it. They often claim to have never even seen the doctor! This is frightening, not only due to the stunning neglect by the M.D., but because they have left their patient at the mercy of a nurse.

Now, I am the first to say that the study of medicine is a noble one, and I have a great deal of respect for most doctors, and for their immense erudition. This is one of the most challenging fields in all of academia to say the least. However, I must defer to what many prominent people have said on the matter for centuries and centuries because they express this sentiment far better than I ever could.

For Instance, Voltaire opined, "Men who are occupied in the restoration of health to other men, by the joint exertion of skill and humanity, are above all the great of the earth." Plato had the most arousing statement when he said, "Medicine requires the knowledge and desires of the body, and how to satisfy them." Henry Louis Meneken quipped, "One of the chief objects of medicine is to save us from the natural consequences of our vices and follies." Clearly, throughout history, physicians have been some of the most highly regarded members of any society. What more could I possibly add?

My last point is only a reminder for doctors and their staff. If you want your patient to have the brand name medication as opposed to the generic, then you have to specifically write "medically necessary" on the rx. No other words will do. You cannot write "brand only" or "brand necessary." At least, this is the case in the state of Florida where I practice.

On my podcast I recounted an argument I had with a doctor that caught the attention of Michael Dean the creator of Freedomtrainonline.com. It must have made an impression because he included my podcast among his family of shows. For a hilarious account of this particularly fascinating exchange I had with Dr. Zod, go to my podcast site www.retailpharmacypodcast.com and search the archives for "Calling Dr. Zod." [9]

---

9   http://web.me.com/jmbovee/Site/Retail_Pharmacy_Podcast/En-tries/2010/4/8_Calling_Dr._Zod.html

Advice for Nurses

"Only two things are infinite, the universe and human stupidity, and I'm not sure about the former."

- Albert Einstein

Only one thing more unnerving than dealing with professionals whose names are followed by a cacophony of letters guaranteeing them a large income and much hubris is their professional brethren who reside more than a few notches lower on the medical-esteem-totem pole. I am referring, of course, to nurses. Before I go any further I have to make a qualifier here. I have friends and family members who are nurses so I take no pleasure in focusing my sites on them, but it must be done nonetheless. Also, I recognize that nurses receive much blame for things that are done by receptionists posing as the real thing. Having said that, let's proceed.

Nurses are a curious group. Part of me has sympathy for them because it cannot be easy dealing with those who assuredly provide a constant reminder to them of their place in the scheme of things. I am sure their inferiority is screeched into them by M.D.s like nails on a chalkboard. In fact, if I had to work all day long with these physicians, I'd probably need treatment for post-traumatic stress disorder. The only problem is when nurses, in a sad attempt to salvage some self-esteem, desperately try to re-inflate their ego by overplaying their hand with pharmacists.

It is one thing dealing with egomaniacal doctors who are a bit abrasive at times, but what excuse do nurses have? They are the surly medical practitioners that Jerry Seinfeld jokes about, but often times lack the intellectual armory to back it up. Most everyone is familiar with the old joke, "What do you call a med school dropout? A dentist." Well...what do you call a pharmacy school dropout? A nurse. While I'm at it, do you know what to call a physical therapy dropout? That's right, a crackerpractor, I mean chiropractor. There's some more medical humor for you.

Pharmacy technicians can often times be grossly incompetent, but at least the pharmacist, by law, is required to hang over them like Gollum did with his "precious." Nurses, on the other hand, will downright guess over the phone when asked about a patient's medication, and the doctor has no idea. Then, come to find out, not only were they way off, but dangerously so. Sometimes, as a pharmacist, you get the impression that they are just making a lot of stuff up as they go. For instance, I cannot tell you how many times I have called simply to find out the doctor's name since his signature was illegible only to have the sig change all of a sudden.

Only an ignoramus would risk guessing about something so vital when the answers are so readily available. There is no excuse when someone's life is potentially on the line and is in their hands. I have busted nurses countless times over the years who were either too busy or too lazy to look up a patient's chart, and instead guessed only to be caught red handed. I only hope that the realization that they may have almost killed someone hit them that night as they put their head to their pillow, and were hit with a severe case of anxiety-induced insomnia.

I have a question for you nurses, why, after I receive a phone message on my IVR authorizing a refill request with additional refills, do I get a fax 45 minutes later for the exact same rx this time with a different number of additional refills? Now I have two rxs for the patient, ostensibly for the same purpose, but with a discrepancy, and then have to spend gobs of time trying to reconcile.

Apparently one of the duties of a nurse is to leave the message on their answering device. For example, the typical nurse's line reading sounds something like this, "You have reached the office of Dr. Dopey, Grumpy, and Sneezy. If this is an emergency dial 911. If you are a patient or pharmacy, please allow for 24 to 48 hours for a response. If you are neither, then why are you calling us? By the way, my name is Janet and I grew up in Boise, Idaho. My parents are Edna and George...." Blah, blah, blah... Just once I want to leave a response saying, "Whew! I began wondering if there was a gas station between me and the end of that message because I was going to have to hit the restroom if that went on much longer. I'm surprised you didn't do five minutes on the weather while you were at it."

All too often they are pretenders with only a rudimentary understanding of what they think they've mastered. Most of them cannot even correctly call in a rx over the phone; a basic duty of theirs I would imagine. Also forgotten in this process of calling in scripts over the phone is breathing. Ladies, please, take a couple of respirations while leaving the message. Too many of you sound like this: "ThisisLindafromDr.Ray'sofficecallinginascriptforpatientMar yNeverminddateofbirth12/3/49,sheneedsgemfibrozil600mgtwobid withfoodandthreerefills..." For Pete's sake ladies, take a breath, and pause at the end of your sentences; that's what periods are for.

I have another question, when I leave a detailed message on your voicemail, why do you call me back without the answer? Far, far too often they will call me back, "Yeah, you had a question about Mr. Johnson's rx?" I respond, "Yes." Then there is silence. I assume they got my message because they did call me back, but apparently I have to re-ask. So after doing so I hear, "Oh, well I don't know. I'll have to get with the doctor and call you back."

Now this is fascinating. She obviously got the message. Did she not listen to all of it? Did she just look at the caller ID and call me back without bothering to listen to it? Why call back without the answer only to have to call me back yet again? What a pointless phone call that was, and what a tremendous waste of time.

Despite the fact that the law requires it, nurses are also stubbornly reluctant to say which M.D. they work under. All too often pharmacists have to call back and say, "Who is the supervising physician for this rx?" Nurses more often than not react angrily and adamantly proudly declaring, "I have the right to call in rxs." They're like Eric Cartman in South Park, "Respect my authority!" I often respond, "Yes, I can see how very proud of yourself you are, but unfortunately I cannot legally fill this rx unless I know who the doctor is. Oh yeah, plus the insurance company won't pay for it without a Drug Enforcement Administration (DEA) number." Sorry ladies, but your license number often times just does not cut it.

Nurses are primarily women. Ever see Meet the Parents or One Flew Over the Cuckoos Nest? It may behoove them to dispatch the stereotype as the Nurse Ratchet type by, well, not being that way. In other words, please extend to us the same professional courtesy we extend to you.

Tips for nurses:

1. S-P-E-L-L-!_!_!

2. S-P-E-L-L-!_!_!

3. S-P-E-L-L-!_!_!

4. Please provide the name of the doctor you work under. We not only need their DEA number, which is required for insurance purposes and helps with our computer search, but the law demands it. We realize that you are proud of your degree, and that you can legally call in rxs. We are not questioning your acumen, we just have to do what we have to do.

5. Please slow down your cadence. When you sound like a tobacco auctioneer pepped up on methamphetamines we have a great deal of trouble writing down everything you say, and do not have the time to replay your entire message 17 times in an effort to jot it all down. Even

then, there is no guarantee that we'll successfully translate. If you have a strong accent, then please spell *everything*, and this goes for those of you who call with a mouth full of food as well.

6. When you call in to our IVR, please tell us up front the number of rxs because when you say, "I'm calling in a prescription for so-and-so," then we use the entire face of the rx pad. Then, when you belatedly say, "...and I also need to call in..." we now have no room on the face of the rx pad and have to scrunch it in.

7. Please do not get angry with us for calling back to verify something. We are simply doing our job. If you had done yours properly, then we would not have to call back. Remember, our first interest is for the patient and their safety.

8. Please do not guess. Take the time to look up the patient's chart, or get with the doctor. We do not mind waiting for accuracy.

Again, I respect all health care providers to the best of my ability, but it is difficult when you have conversations such as the following:

Me: "I am calling to verify a controlled rx because the month and quantity were not written in textual format."

Nurse: "What does that mean 'textual format'?"

Me: "It means that it has to be written out in letters."

Nurse: "What do you mean by, 'It has to be written out in letters?'"

Me: "You know letters...the things we use to make the alphabet. I cannot possibly say it any more simply."

Advice for Pharmacists

"Society's demands for moral authority and character increase as the importance of the position increases."

- John Adams

Every pharmacist has their own way of doing things. Despite this, there are still some standard practices shared between all retail pharmacies everywhere. Conversely, there are some practices that are inappropriate despite the setting as well. Following are some of the more common examples.

Transfers from another pharmacy are typically a 24-hour wait, especially during 'season'. Sure, it doesn't necessarily take that long, but it is an indeterminate amount of time. We give this time frame because it guarantees it will be ready when we say it will. Some pharmacists will try to do them immediately, and more often than not they'll pull it off; however, on those few occasions when the other pharmacy's phone is busy, they never answer the phone, they keep placing you on hold for an exceedingly long time, ask that you call back later, or even hang up on you, then you set yourself up for the curmudgeon who intones, "What?! You mean it isn't ready yet? But you told me it would only take 15 minutes!" Those customers are why most pharmacies make transfers a standard 24-hour transaction.

When you have to order a drug for a patient, you tell them the day it will be in, but tell them the time as well. All too often a patient will either call or show up just as we are opening the pharmacy expecting to get their rx. Even if you receive your order in the morning, you still have to give yourself time for unpredictable circumstances. What if your tech calls in sick or is late? What if the delivery is late? What if you are unusually busy the next morning? The point is to give yourself a cushion of a few hours. So, if your order comes in around 10 a.m., then tell the patients that their rxs will be ready around 2 p.m., or even 4 p.m.

We will either call or fax the doctor's office for refills, but if it is a new rx, then we usually tell the customer we cannot. Why is that? One reason is because if it is a new rx, then there is nothing we can print to fax to the doctor's office. We can either call the office, tell them what the patient wants, and let them call it in as a new rx, or the patient can give the doctor's office our fax or phone number, and tell them to contact us. Typically, if it has been a long time since the patient was seen by the doctor, he or she will want to see the patient before calling in a rx. Once the customer is established in our system, and has been on the drug before, then this is not necessary.

I had a partner once who would give customers a hard time when they came up and asked where specific over-the-counter (OTC) items were. His reply would be, "Where have you looked so far?" You see, he resented the fact that they would immediately come right up asking where something was without trying to look for it on their own first. This, however, only prolongs the conversation. I recommend, at the minimum, at least rattling off the isle number where it is, and which side of the isle it is on. Ideally, the OTC stock person, or your tech will show them where the item is.

As described earlier, due to the increasing frequency of third party PA rejections, pharmacists are now refusing to even make those calls (as are doctors as well). Some pharmacists actually tell the patient to call the doctor, and tell him or her to call their insurance company, thus leaving it entirely in their hands. This is where I draw the line.

The average patient has no idea what a PA is, and despite how clearly and frequently you explain it to them, they seldom understand it. They'll nod their head and pretend, and then two hours later you will get an angry call from the doctor's nurse asking indignantly why you refused to give the patient their medicine. Sigh... Do everyone a favor, and just make that call. Doctors are more and more refusing to do it, but that is no reason for us to refuse to help their patients.

Now, I am not an angel, okay? I confess that when a patient gets pushy with the wait time for their rx, I may tend to go even slower. Ever see that bumper sticker, "The closer you get, the slower I drive?" Same thing goes here. This is not a power trip, as you may think. No, this is customer training.

You do not want people thinking that they can pull certain stunts every time they come in to the pharmacy. It is a very good precedent to establish, right off of the bat, what behavior you deem intolerable. It sounds condescending, but people need training, and if you work a lot of overtime at other pharmacies, then you can certainly tell the difference between pharmacies where pharmacists subscribe to this creed and where they do not.

I recently had a woman drop off her refill, and then stand at the counter waiting for it. I was on the phone with another patient's insurance company trying to get approval on a rx claim. This woman could clearly see that I was engaged in a previous endeavor. Still she stood there. I told her it may be a while. She responded, "You're not busy. I always get it in about 10 minutes." Choking on my own rage, I could not vocalize a reply. I simply widened my eyes in utter disbelief, and turned my back on her. She got the message. Yes, I know, not terribly professional, but we are human too, and I was disgusted.

First of all, who the heck are you to tell me how busy I am? Unless you have worked retail pharmacy yourself, then how would you know? I was alone at the time, and had a lot to do. Just because there's no crowd in front of the pharmacy does not mean there aren't several people shopping in the store who have dropped their rxs off way ahead of you who will be back soon for pick up.

It also never occurred to this woman that some times and some days are busier than others. Did she honestly believe it would always be 10 minutes each and every single time she came in? Does it never dawn on customers that pharmacies increase their business from when they first open, and get busier and busier over time, and in certain seasons?

The selling of syringes is a prime example where customer training is vital. Drug addicts overrun pharmacies where they are sold without any compunction. Again, watch Don't Shoot the Pharmacist. I have to admit that every so often it is amusing to hear them make up stories as to why they need needles. The sympathetic character of choice is usually the grandmother. Sometimes it is for their dog, or other such pet. These people learn very quickly, by word of mouth, not to come to my pharmacy.

The same goes for the oxycodone seekers, which are legion in Florida. Be sure to always have some hand sanitizer nearby after touching anything they hand to you, and perhaps a germ filter mask. I swear each and every one of them smells like they just got off from a 48-hour shift in a Marlboro factory. Either that or they were trapped in someone's windowless basement while their captive was holding a two-week cigar convention. For a more in depth look at the oxycodone epidemic see the appendix. (Appendix G)

They say you shouldn't judge a book by its cover, but whoever said that did not work retail. In our business you have to. I let it be clearly known that no drug addicts will get any syringes from me. Other pharmacists say that if we do not, then we just force them to share needles, and thus spread disease. There was a drug addict who actually had the gall to threaten this course of action after I refused to sell syringes to him. That threat holds no sway over me. I will not be an enabler of that lifestyle. I am also offended at their lack of effort and originality in trying to fool me. I mean really, how far do they think they are going to get coming in looking like Jay and Silent Bob with a hangover?

Inevitably, one pharmacist will ask their partner to switch days for some reason. Maybe your partner needs a day off, and is out of vacation time. When I was Assistant Pharmacy Manager, the Pharmacy Manager would not only ask me to work for her on a specific day, but would tell me what day she would work for me in return. Do not go along with this. They are the one who needs a favor from you. They are the one who need you to work a specific day for them. Why should they also get to choose what day they will work for you? When this is requested of me I simply say, "Let me deposit the day that you owe me in the bank, and when the time comes when I require a specific day off, then I'll let you know that I need to make a withdrawal." Now, that is true equality.

It is crucial that you get along with your partner, and that you two stay in contact so that you are on the same page. This is why we are required to overlap at least once a week. I have not always been terribly fortunate in this area, but rather than write a 500-page chapter on Partners, I'll dedicate much of the next book on this subject.

One thing I cannot stress enough is, train your techs, and do not allow them to run rampant doing as they please, otherwise they will remain untrained and unhelpful. Make your expectations clear to them and post their daily duties on the bulletin board if necessary. For a basic list of opening and closing tech duties see the appendix. (Appendix H)

Do not allow lazy techs to get away with willful ignorance. Evaluate them honestly, make fair criticisms, specify particular things they need to improve on, and document everything. Once enough time has passed, you have done everything you could to help them, and no improvement has been made, then you have enough documentation to back your decision to remove them from your pharmacy.

My most important piece of advice for pharmacists is to document everything. If you have a bad apple as a tech, or partner, and you want to get them out of your pharmacy, then you had better have a stack of evidence (or ammunition as I see it) to back up your contentions. You need to show a consistent pattern of poor customer service with written complaints by your patients. You need to show laziness or incompetence with printouts indicating how long it takes the person in question to fill a rx, or type one up, or how few they fill on their days. You need to be able to show the condition they leave the pharmacy when you come in on your mornings. You need testimony from other staff either in the pharmacy, or even in other departments.

Write down specifics with dates, and even times. Write down names of people and what they said. The two worst pharmacists I have ever seen were not only lazy and incompetent, were not only messy and disorganized, but they were downright cruel to everyone in the store including the customers.

I can only go by my own personal experiences here, obviously, but the floaters that I have had to deal with have been nightmarish. Invariably, what happens when you come in the day after (think nuclear blast) these subs have defiled your pharmacy involves: massive clean up, total re-organization, the solving of many mysteries, the search for lost items, the filling of many rxs that should have been filled during their shift, and incessant apologizing to a seemingly never ending cacophony of disgruntled customers who had the sad misfortune of suffering the abuses of these dopes.

I would complain to my supervisor about them and suggest that they perhaps be re-trained since none of them seemed able to do the most rudimentary tasks, but as per usual my pleas fell upon deaf ears. A couple of floaters actually called me the day before their reign, and would ask about the tech help they would be provided. Whenever I said that we had no tech, the panic would set in and they'd proclaim, "I don't do the register." In the appendix I have a note that I posted in my pharmacy for the floaters who I had to endure for such a long time, and who were tearing my pharmacy up on a daily basis. (Appendix I)

Lastly, after making this error myself I have learned to not hassle my supervisor with micro-management, or minor issues. I am convinced that the primary reason Zap had it in for me was because I was a thorn in his side too frequently begging him to resolve some issue. True, I was on an amazing run of bad luck because of the stupendous jerks I had to deal with, solely his own doing, but despite that I now realize that I was digging my own grave by bugging him so often. He also clearly did not like my political views, a subject which he would bring up mind you, but surely no one deserves to be persecuted for their politics (insert sarcasm).

I have said it before and I will say it again, we are surrounded by crazy, stupid people. Pharmacists, despite their excellent reputation, also suffer from bad apples, and it continues to get worse with time. If this persists, we will one day be ranked down there with lawyers, politicians, and car salesmen as some of the least trusted professionals in the country on the next Pew research poll.

Advice for Dealing With Pharmacy Supervisors

"It's important to let people know what you stand for. It's equally important that they know what you won't stand for."

- B. Bader

Allow me to preface this chapter by first saying that I have never and will never seek the role as Pharmacy Supervisor. When one considers how much more responsibility, stress, and bologna one has to put up with for the slight increase in pay…it is simply not worth it. Having said that, if you take on that responsibility, then you had better be prepared to do it right. So far, I have worked under four supervisors, and am currently two for four. Funny, the two that I got along with, and who liked me, were employed by the same company.

The first one hired me fresh out of school, and was somewhat unpopular, but I liked him and am still friends with him to this day. I once asked him if being a supervisor was "worth it." In short, his answer was, "Not really." He complained that much of his time was spent performing tedious payroll duties. This is pretty much what I had imagined the case to be. Six months after I asked him this, he resigned his position and is now a pharmacy manager.

My next boss was not a bad person, but certainly two-faced. This guy, after receiving a complementary email from a customer about the terrific customer service received, actually sent out a mass email saying that customer complements, "…ought to be genuine and not encouraged." That is simply remarkable, and very sad. Oh, and it also represents terrible leadership brought on by a cynical and unjustified mistrust. You see, this occurred years after I had already quit the company so there is no bias here.

Then I worked for a total doofus, Zap Branigan. He was more of a snake oil salesman than a pharmacy supervisor. He would simply shift bad apples from one pharmacy to another, and point B was often my store. I aged horribly during the two years I worked for him due to his stunningly poor judgment and apathy. Honestly, I had trouble sleeping, my eyes began twitching, and health actually suffered. He was a former bodybuilder who looked like Mr. Incredible during his retirement years when I worked for him.

He was also the only person to ever fire me. I failed to report two simultaneous QREs. It is law that whoever discovers them has the duty to report them as soon as they are realized. Mine were waiting for me the following morning, and I assumed that my partner had already written them up. I should have known better; never assume. However, upon reflection, it is now clear that he had it in for me for quite a while, and was working diligently in this endeavor.

I was a bug buzzing around his ears always complaining about the psychopaths he stuck me with, and he methodically put the pieces in place for the eventual checkmate. Another big mistake I made was failing to realize that the company records and monitors our phone calls. See, I offered my former partner advice as to whether or not she should file a sexual harassment lawsuit against him. I answered in the affirmative.

She explained to me at the time that if you were not inside his circle of cronies, then you were outside, and that did not bode well. He coaxed her into transferring out of our pharmacy, and, after she discovered the ruse, would not allow her to return despite the fact that I had also lobbied for it. He actually had the nerve to use me as his excuse by telling her that I did not want to be demoted upon her return. That was a bald-faced lie. I did not want to be the pharmacy manager at the time.

Obviously, he was the worst supervisor I ever had. He would actually blame me, and others, for his screw-ups. He even did this to his right hand man (our scheduler), who would often concede to his enormous faults and lack of supervisory skill. Zap got on both of us once because no floaters were scheduled for Mr. Magoo's vacation two weeks after being hired.

Mr. Magoo was a grumpy old man who replaced the assistant pharmacist who I refer to on my podcast as Norman Bates. Magoo was horribly inept. It would regularly take him 30 minutes just to type up a single rx into the computer. He also had an Irish temper that made Bill O'Reilly look like Mr. Rogers.

Stunningly, he was just as bad as Norman who once threatened an older woman at our pharmacy with physical violence after taking pictures of her with his camera shouting, "Not only do I know where you live, but now what you look like!" After this guy was finally fired, he performed a scorched earth policy on every retail pharmacy company in southwest Florida, and just as he had done before, eventually had to leave the state to find employment. I performed a more thorough background check on this nut with a five minute Google search than Zap had done over several years time. I found out all sorts of horrible things this guy did before coming to my store including the chaos he caused at the previous store Zap had him assigned to.

As if that ordeal wasn't bad enough, Mr. Magoo raised the bar. Here was yet another total nincompoop that Zap stuck me with. It was like being hit by asshole lightning twice in the same week! One of our customers described him well while complaining to me about him when she said he was, "totally vacant and completely rude."

Well, if the supervisor hires a guy and tells him he may take a week long vacation immediately after his training, then who's fault is it other than the supervisor who hired him? Especially since he did not inform his buddy the scheduler, or me about it. He even got on my case once because I would not drive to the pharmacy during a hurricane; and it wasn't even my day to work!

The floater had also decided life was more important than work, and refused to drive to the store. I was in constant contact with the guy, and he told me as soon as the winds died down he would go to my pharmacy. Why I got chewed out for this is beyond me, but I ended up driving a total of one hour for two hours of actual work time before the floater finally showed up.

Oddly enough, Magoo and I were hired at practically the exact same time by the company I presently work for. We were both brought on as floaters, and I found myself in a familiar position. While working at a pharmacy the day after he was there I had to clean up his messes. After a year and a half, he has yet again, been fired.

Needless to say, Zap was a real gem. In the two years I worked for him I called in sick two and one-half days. His responses to me were exactly the same ones I received when I called in sick as a grocery stock boy, "When did you know this?" As if I can predict when I will be ill. He even tried the old trick of asking, "Can you go in for just a couple of hours?" Then he would call me all throughout the day to make sure I was *really* bedridden. Here I am a doctor in one the most highly respected and trusted professions in the country, and I am being treated like a minimum wage earning schlep. I should have called human resources and reported him.

At this point in my career I was beginning to wonder if pharmacy supervisors were required to be deceitful, vengeful, two-faced ignoramuses that would make your average Washington D.C. politician wince. However, I then went back to where I started, and currently work for an outstanding woman who is always upbeat, and extremely helpful. She actually cares about micro issues such as tech problems, and can still sympathize with us who remain at the front lines, so to speak.

I actually believe that what comes out of her mouth is sincere. Also, I know she reads my emails because she responds to them and does not act like it is the first time I have mentioned something when it is actually my third attempt. I hope to continue to work for her for years to come; I only hope she doesn't get promoted anytime soon.

The company I presently work for is all about customer service. This is understandable because, after all, this is a business. The only time it seems to go too far is when we as pharmacists are told that we need to be more polite to the illicit druggies coming in for syringes, or more courteous to the oxycodone doctor shoppers. I get the impression that they want me to act as if I were a greeter at Disney World or something. At times, pharmacists have to be discerning, and may even have to tell problem customers that they may be better served elsewhere. Sadly, most company supervisors will not condone this or back up their pharmacists who deem it necessary during those rare times. Before long pharmacists confronted by violent drug addicts are going to have to say, "Thank you for not killing us. Please come again!"

Advice for Dealing With Grocery Personnel

"Educated men are as much superior to uneducated men as the living are to the dead."

- Aristotle

At some point, there will be a clash between the pharmacy department manager and at least one or more of the grocery department managers; it is as inevitable as death and taxes. This is especially true in a supermarket setting. The conventional wisdom is that grocery managers deeply resent pharmacy managers because these kids, fresh out of school who are new to the company, often times start out making more than this middle aged company man who has had to work his way up over the past 25 years to get where he is. This may be true, but why blame us? They ought to blame themselves. Then again, I have never understood the impulse to resent those who have things better than I do. Rather, I always think to myself, "Good for them."

Another big issue actually involves the tech. Although their job title is "Pharmacy Technician" and they are under the pharmacy department's payroll, sometimes the grocery department will attempt to commandeer them for the purpose of running a cash register or stocking grocery merchandise. This is a problem because the entire purpose of having a tech in your pharmacy is so that they will help you fill rxs. Their role is not to stock frozen food, or gather shopping carts from the parking lot. Their role is to reduce the number of interruptions, and help prevent it from getting too busy and hectic, all of which increase the likelihood of QREs.

Here are a few points one must make to grocery managers who either do not understand how it works, or are purposefully overstepping the line. First, while they may have say over the meat, deli, produce, grocery department, et al., they really have little influence in the pharmacy department. The pharmacist is the manager of this department, and our duty is to the state and federal laws first, the state board second, our oath to our patients and profession next, and then the company we work for.

Second, people need their medicine in a timely and accurate manner, not their Fruity Pebbles and Cheerios. If the grocery cashier makes a mistake because she's being rushed, then what's the worst thing that will happen- the customer gets their Fruit Loops rung up twice? If we make an error due to hurrying or suffering from too many distracting interruptions, then someone could get hurt or worse. Also, our licenses are on the line back here, and we worked pretty damn hard to get them.

This goes for customer complaints as well. The company I presently work for has the pharmacy supervisor and store manager share in the evaluation of the pharmacy manager. At times, store managers have told me that they have received some customer complaints about me, and that I need to work on my customer service skills. However, there is a difference between customer complaints vis-à-vis the pharmacy department versus other departments.

As someone who is beholden to the law, I often times have to tell patients things they do not want to hear. I am required, at times, to say "No" and refuse to do what is being requested of me. For instance, I cannot sell syringes to someone if I deem them to be using them for illicit drug use. I cannot fill an oxycodone, or any other CII narcotic rx, if I do not feel it is for a legitimate medical purpose. I cannot fax 50 sheets of paper for a single customer, especially for a non-pharmacy related purpose. This is a pharmacy, not a Kinkos. I cannot refill a rx too soon for cash just because the patient wants me to if it is clear they are abusing the respective drug.

In addition, we are dealing with colorful customers many of whom have a variety of disorders such as bipolar disorder, major depressive disorder, severe anxiety disorder, etc. Some people have all of the above. So when our pharmacy customers come in not only are they not feeling particularly well, not only have they just endured an unpleasant ordeal at the doctor's office, not only are their medical, dental, or prescription insurance plans refusing to pay for their services and drugs, but many of them are simply nutters. A customer complaining that the bakery ran out of wheat bread is not the same thing.

There is no equivalency between the pharmacy and other grocery departments. Grocery customers do not suffer physically and emotionally if they have to wait longer; well, physically any way. Basically, our customers have to be there involuntarily. They come because they are either in severe pain, have an infection, have AIDS or cancer, or are just plain ill. They do not want to wait one minute longer than they have to, and they shouldn't.

I cannot recall how many times I have called for just one of the many grocery cashiers to come help me at a busy time only to get a surly remark like, "Well, we're busy too. Can't you ring up your own prescriptions?" This level of insubordination is remarkable. The pharmacy manager is still a manager in the store, and for a cashier to make such a quip is inexcusable. Of course, when the grocery managers hold you in the same regard, then what is to be expected?

I actually had one tell me that, "You're not doing enough business. You should be more like the sushi department and cut back." I replied, "But I have no techs. There is no one to cut back on." "Well, you need to cut back your operating hours," she insisted. Mind you, this was an assistant grocery manager, and it was her first day in our store. Also, as far as I know, she has no authority whatsoever to demand, or even suggest, such a thing. Now, is it only I, or is it not innately insane to say that the pharmacy department needs to be more like the sushi department? How many doctors work in the other departments?

This same person once gave me a look that would have turned Medusa into stone when I asked her if there was a bagger or stock boy who could hang our banner outside the store advertising our flu shots. Apparently she expected me to go to the back room, grab a ladder, grab the banner, walk outside (which is forbidden by law), hang the banner myself, and then return the ladder. Remember now, I had no tech help at the time, so who was going to watch the pharmacy while I did all of this?

She once said to me, as I was returning from the restroom, "Hey Jean-Marc, your pharmacy phone has been ringing off the hook." My reply was, "Well there's no bathroom in the pharmacy, and I can't bring the phone with me, so what do you want me to do?" It's not like I was just walking around socializing like grocery personnel do oh so often. I was on my way back to the pharmacy, after all, and am working a 12-hour shift with no breaks.

So our phone monitor not only wanted me to hang banners outside, but after I tried to take two sleeves of regular 8 X 11 plain white paper from the manager's office for our printer, and she stopped dead in her tracks and said, "Why don't you order your own paper?" I said it was because whenever I do I never see it because no one ever brings it to us. "Well go in the back and look for it," was her reply.

This is the same person who is ever so concerned about my phone ringing when I'm in the John. She is also the same person who I was told by my boss to allow back behind the pharmacy counter so that she could fax her own stuff because, "It's a good way to build bridges." I wanted to tell Mrs. Build Bridges To, "Listen, why don't you go to pharmacy school for 6 years, pass, take your two state board exams, pass those, get certified in MTM, CPR, and flu shot administration, and then you can cover the pharmacy for me while

I'm hanging banners outside and traipsing through the backroom for my paper."

She once said to me that the pharmacy department is responsible for how we are looked upon and prejudiced against. Apparently, according to her, the pharmacist who worked at her previous location tried to put her in her place by pointing out the difference in their education level. While it seems arrogant to do so, you have to realize that he probably did it to get her off of his back. Sadly, I think all he did was build upon her shoulder the chip that she has regarding the pharmacy department.

I once had an egomaniacal office cashier regularly refuse to release the only clerk in the entire store who was HIPPA trained, and thus able to help me in the pharmacy. I would page for assistance over the intercom system, and she would peek over, see that there was no crowd at the pharmacy, and thus make the self-determination that, "Ah, he doesn't need any help." As if she were qualified to make that determination.

She even took it upon herself once to declare that, "From this day hence forth all rxs will be rung up in the pharmacy department only, and no longer in the grocery department." Fortunately it was not long before the store manager overruled her, but what gall, eh? She thought she could rule the place like frickin' Caesar, or something; however, the only throne I can see her on may be a hemorrhoid cushion.

Grocery people often fail to realize that we are paid for mostly mental work. This is why we get cranky when interrupted, or harassed about what we regard to be frivolities. Traditionally, people who sit get paid more than people who stand, and there is a reason for that. Most grocery personnel lack the erudition to comprehend exactly what it is that we do, what is going on in our minds, and what we have to put up with.

In any case, when both departments are busy, the pharmacist needs to make it clear that the tech stays. If you work at a slow store it is harder to convince the grocery personnel because they so often see you and your tech sitting around not doing much. Remind them that even slow pharmacies have busy moments, and even if you are not busy at the moment, you could be busy at any moment.

Thirdly, grocery managers have to understand that not only do they have little to no say in what goes on in the pharmacy, but they have even less authority over you. In fact, if they are not HIPPA trained, then they are not even permitted to enter your pharmacy. They cannot force you to fill any rx that you do not want to fill, for whatever reason, and they especially cannot take your tech away from you, unless you allow them to. They are gagging how much of a pushover you are. As discussed previously, even your very own techs will try this from time to time.

Case in point, this assistant manager once told me I had to be at the store at 5 AM for inventory. Traditionally it has always been no earlier than 6 AM. I doubt that there is a pharmacist on the entire North American continent who shows up for inventory at 5 AM. I chuckled and said, "When that order comes from my supervisor, then I'll be there."

Not to put too fine a point on it, but we had a brief argument once about the company clock that hangs in my pharmacy. I wanted to write up two double-a batteries and charge them to the pharmacy department, and she said, "I think you ought to pay for that out of your own pocket." I replied, "This is a company clock! I'd just as soon throw it in the trash before I pay out of pocket for the batteries." She hesitated, but then finally relented.

You should handle these situations responsibly, but that does not mean you have to cave in to them. Hopefully, your supervisor will back you up. This is not solely because they were once in your shoes, but because they fully understand that you have the right to draw the line, professionally. Eighty percent of supervisors do not want to be troubled with trifles, but in straightening out the minds of the grocery staff, you may require their assistance.

There was only one time a pharmacy supervisor did not back me (guess who). I once had a store manager commandeer my tech, and had her go outside to gather shopping carts from the parking lot. Naturally, I protested stating how ludicrous it was to steal my one and only helper when the grocery department had dozens of employees at their disposal. His response was, "Hey, if I can do it, then she can do it." Well, there is no mention of "cart gathering" in any pharmacy technician's job description.

Once I saw that his ego was preventing the rationality of my argument from piercing through, I then resorted to my supervisor-slash-snake oil salesman Zap for help. After explaining the situation to him, his astonishing response was, "Do you have a problem with that?" I was speechless. Yes I did, in fact.

No tech should ever be commandeered by the grocery department to go outside to retrieve shopping carts. It is simply not a part of their job. Even his lackey, our scheduler, was incredulous when I told him about it. Unbeknownst to me, this was par for the course at this particular company. Now that I look back, Zap was the cause of most of the problems I have encountered in my retail pharmacy career. Thank goodness he fired me; I might still be working there currently hating my job, and life in general, if it were not for his personal dislike of me.

The grocery manager at this particular store also had the Health, Beauty, & Cosmetics (HBC) stock girl, who was under the pharmacy department's payroll, stocking various grocery items from day one, and despite being alarmed by that, Zap did nothing about it…surprise, surprise. This company was largely a last stop for drunkards and incompetents on their last resort, and also a retirement community for elderly folks whose arms and legs move slow, and whose minds move even slower, which explains my "20 Year" tech. I'll never forget what it was like working with her. It was like being stuck in yet another George Romero movie-The Walking Brain Dead.

In some ways she, and many of the employees there, were like zombies with barren eyes, and a chimpanzee-like attention to detail. Just a bunch of intellectually herniated diamond-studded dimwits who were not just diaphanous, but were constantly engaged in weapons grade banality and museum quality insipidness. That is my homage to Dennis Miller.

Real Life Retail Pharmacy Conversations

"Never underestimate the power of human stupidity"

- Robert Heinlein

This chapter is just for fun. I want to show some of the bizarre conversations we pharmacists have to engage in from time to time. Admittedly, these are some of the stranger ones, but they are illustrative of the point I often make about our deserving of honorary degrees in sociology.

Too many people fail to think before they talk. Rather than elaborate too deeply on this point, allow me to provide a prime example of an honest to God real conversation I had with a woman at my counter once.

Me: *"Such and such* Pharmacy, this is the pharmacist. How may I help you?"

Patient: "Hello?"

Me: "Yes, *such and such* Pharmacy, pharmacist speaking. How may I help you?"

Patient: "Is this the pharmacy?"

Me: "Yyyess..."

Patient: "Are you the pharmacist?"

Me: [sigh] "Yes."

Patient: "You're the pharmacist?"

Me: [-------]

Patient: "Hello? I need a drug."

Me: "You need a refill?"

Patient: "No, I need my heart drug."

Me: "Okay, so you need a refill on your heart drug. Um, what is your name?"

Patient: "[incredibly complex name, then long pause]"

Me: "..............would you like to spell that for me?"

Patient: "[mumbly letters flying at light speed]"

Me: "Okay, Mrs. Supercalifragilistic, what is your date of birth?"

Patient: "Why do you need that?!"

Me: "It helps me find you in the computer."

Patient: "six-nine-five"

Me: "No, your date of birth."

Patient: "Huh?"

Me: "You called to refill a drug. I need to know which one it is."

Patient: "I said, my heart medicine!"

Me: [beginning to sob] "Yeah, but here's the problem, you have several heart meds."

Patient: "hydra...hydrolo...hydralozazine?"

Me: "Hydrochlorothiazide? Okay, no problem."

Patient: "Hello?"

Me: [really tearing up now] "Yes, no problem, we'll get it ready."

Patient: "How long will it take?"

Me: "About a half-hour."

Patient: "That long?! I have a plane to catch in less than an hour. Are you serious?!"

Me: "Are you?" [internally screaming in disbelief]

Now, believe it or not, that is not an uncommon conversation. Every pharmacist gets one of these periodically. However, there is absolutely no need for the following real life conversation.

Me: "Mr. Johnson, your insurance rejected your prescription."

Patient: "What do you mean?! Why?!"

Me: "It says 'NDC Not Covered', they don't cover this drug anymore."

Patient: "Well why the hell not?! They have *before*! My insurance is still good! That's incorrect."

Me: "Uh huh, well you may want to call them and find out why. Only they can tell you what is..."

Interrupting Patient: "Why can't you tell me?"

Me: "Because I'm not your insurance. Only they know..."

Interrupting Patient: "Well, I'll be damned if I'm gonna pay for it!"

Me: "So, would me like me to hold it for now?"

Patient: "No! I want you to sell it to me for my co-pay!"

Me: "But your insurance..."

Interrupting Patient: "Oh, that's bullshit! You're scamming me!"

Me: "Yeah, that's what we do here."

Patient: "I know how much profit you guys make!"

Me: "Actually the pharmacy doesn't make much..."

Interrupting Patient: "Bullshit!"

Me: "Sir, is there anything else I can help you with?"

Patient: "Yeah! I want you to explain to me why you won't give me my medicine!"

Me: "I've already explained everything. I can't simplify it any further for you. You can still get your medicine. You just have to pay cash."

Patient: "But it was covered the last time."

Me: "Yes, I see that, but something has obviously changed since then. I suggest that you call your insurance. They will answer all of your questions."

Usually, at this point the customer gives you a blank stare for several seconds before walking off in disgust. What follows is a short exchange I had with a woman while I was writing this book.

Patient: "Where's your ice cream?"

Me: "I don't know. In the frozen food section?"

Patient: "You work here don't you?"

Me: "In the pharmacy. I don't stock ice cream."

Patient: "Ice cream in the pharmacy?!"

Me: "Exactly."

Communicating with foreigners is difficult for the obvious reasons such as the language barrier, but some people seem to need special help. The following exchange was between myself and a Haitian woman who just seemed completely confused.

Haitian woman at counter just staring at me:

JM: "Yes ma'am."

Haitian woman: "I need prescription."

JM: "You're here to pick up a prescription?"

Haitian woman: "Yes."

JM: "What is the last name?"

Haitian woman: "Blanter."

After not finding anything I say: "Blanter? I don't see anything for Blanter. That's B as in 'boy'?"

Haitian woman: "Yes. Blanter."

After failing a second time she asked for the rx back. When I finally found it I saw that the last name was Planter. I said, "B as in boy!" Despite the fact that it was now found, she was upset about the $50 co-pay, and wanted the rx back. She was also angry because the drug had to be ordered yesterday when she first dropped off the rx with my partner, and the order had not come in yet; it was only 10 a.m. Later in the day she came back with the rx in hand and wanted it filled. I said it would be about twenty minutes, and she became angry all over again. She expected it to still be ready, but I had to rescan the rx, type it up all over, and fill it yet again. When it was all said and done, she signed her name with an 'X.'

Another Haitian woman came in to pick up an albuterol rx. After she got home she called to say she received the wrong drug, and that she wanted the metformin instead. I told her that she said albuterol when she called it in and again at the pick up window, and so that is what I gave her. She insisted she said metformin so I agreed to do an exchange. When she came back I handed her the metformin and she said she did not want it. She now wanted the albuterol. Astonished, I said, "That is what I gave you the first time," and then I stared at her in stunned silence. As if that wasn't bad enough, the next day a Haitian man did the same exact thing. Mental note - stay the hell away from the Haitian rum that I see in the liquor section of my store.

Once I had a gay couple come in, and it was their first visit. The one gentleman's rx was rejected by his insurance because it was a refill too soon. After I explained this relatively simple thing to him, his life partner indignantly barked, "You're going to let him go without his medicine?!" Shocked, I responded, "Huh?" Then the man who's rx was rejected said, "My doctor will just have to call it in." I then explained, "No, that will not make any difference. It is not that you do not have a valid rx here, it is just that the insurance thinks it is too soon to fill it again. They think you should still have plenty left for now."

His reply was, "Are you saying my doctor will let me go without my medication?!" At this point I'm thinking, "What?!" So I replied, "I did not say that. You can always pay cash, and get it right now." The term "cash" threw him off. "Cash?! Don't you accept credit cards? That is all I have with me!" At this point I'm looking at them wondering if they are putting me on, or are these guys actually this thin skinned and stupid. I answered, "By the term "cash" I mean out of pocket, not through the insurance. 'Cash' includes credit or debit cards."

There was actually a time when an older gentleman was yelling at me because he went to one of our other stores and they did not have amoxicillin. I thought that was odd because what pharmacy runs out of amoxicillin? It turns out that he thought it was over the counter, and went to one of our stores that did not have a pharmacy.

I had to explain to him, "Sir, that is a prescription drug. You have to get it at a pharmacy. The reason you couldn't find it is because you went to a store that had no pharmacy." All I received in return was a blank stare. Perhaps it is patients like these that account for the poor attitude and rude demeanor of so many receptionists who call us from doctor's offices since I imagine these people probably spread joy everywhere they go.

Patients and other health care professionals are not the only ones who provide migraine-inducing conversations. What follows is an exchange between an insurance company receptionist and myself. I can only imagine how it will be once universal health care passes, and we have to deal with government employees.

JM: "Yes, I am getting a 'date of birth' rejection on a claim."

Ins. Agent: "The patient's name?"

JM: "Lizbeth Kooky-Guevera. No 'E' at the beginning."

Ins. Agent: "The ID number and date of birth?"

JM: "########, 1/3/53."

Ins. Agent: "I'm not finding her…Elizabeth?"

JM: "There's no E at beginning."

Ins. Agent: "The date of birth?"

JM: "1/3/53."

Then she places me on hold. Another agent answers and I have to start from scratch. Perhaps it was her first day. Later that same day I had to call the local VA Clinic for a rx transfer. I had to call twice because I was disconnected after the first call. What follows is a look at our future.

JM: "This is Marc at *such and such* pharmacy. I need a transfer."

VA Receptionist: "We at the VA don't do transfers."

JM: "Do you have a pharmacy there?"

VA Receptionist: "Yes."

JM: "Can you please transfer me to the pharmacy?"

After finally getting through to a pharmacist, I was told that the rx could not be transferred.

JM: "Well then can I at least get the doctor info?"

VA Pharmacist: "What do you want?"

JM: "The doctor's phone number."

VA Pharmacist: "Why?"

JM: "So I can get a new rx for the patient and then fill it."

VA Pharmacist: "He has plenty of refills here."

JM: "But he's not there, we're in Florida, and you just told me you can't transfer them."

VA Pharmacist: "Well I can send them to you."

JM: "You just told me u don't do transfers. Is that a new law in Rhode Island?"

VA Pharmacist: "Yes, but we can put you through to our tap line."

JM: "What's that?"

VA Pharmacist: "It will connect you to the doctor."

Now that is a cumbersome process. Transferring rxs takes long enough, but this was a new one for me. Thankfully, I have not had to call any Rhode Island VA Clinics since.

Here's a conversation Abbott and Costello would love. While standing at the pick up window a man approaches me:

Me: "Yes sir. Are you dropping off?"

Mr. Confused: "No, not really." Then he hands me two rxs.

Me: "That's dropping off. This is the *pick up* window. Let's go down to the drop off window because it is only there that I can scan and input the rxs."

Mr. Confused: "I thought you meant 'drop off' and then come back."

Me: "I meant 'drop off'. That was pick up. By the way, who is on first?"

Really now, the signs were in English. This was an English speaking Caucasian man. I was speaking clear English. Perhaps he was just listening in dingbat. This reminds me of a study done recently showing that one in five Americans, or nearly 45 million people, suffer from mental illness. [10] From my personal daily observations it seems more like four out of five.

10   http://www.physorg.com/news/2010-11-americans-mental-illness-year-survey.html

The Future of Retail Pharmacy

"Soap and water, and common sense are the best disinfectants."

- William Osler

The art of practicing retail pharmacy has changed drastically over the last ten years, and continues to. In point of fact, it has changed so much that a survey conducted by Drug Topics Magazine in their May 19, 2010 edition showed that 46% of pharmacists would not encourage their son or daughter to pursue a career in pharmacy. It causes at least one eyebrow to rise upon the realization that nearly half of all pharmacists would purposefully steer their own kids in another direction away from their own profession.

It started with George Bush's passing of the Medicare Prescription Drug Modernization Act, which provided help in the purchasing of prescription medications for 40 million of our senior citizens at the price of over $1 trillion. It was the largest expansion of Medicare since the program was created in 1965. In addition to the prescription drug benefits, the measure provided billions of dollars in subsidies to insurance companies and health maintenance organizations. High on the list of things not covered in the bill was a mechanism to stem rising prescription drug costs, but it was believed that competition would be the remedy for that. To some extent, it shifted retail pharmacy reimbursement from cash to third-party transactions, and complicated the entire process of filling rxs. [11]

The next deleterious factor was the economic downturn that began in 2008. As a result, companies began looking for ways to cut operating costs, and increase business. Many pharmacies began to offer flu shots, MTM, cheaper generics, 90 day supply plans, free antibiotics, free diabetes drugs, etc. Almost universally practiced in the retail pharmacy world was a movement toward central filling, where pharmacists at a central location help type up rxs and resolve third party issues for other pharmacies. This led to the slashing of tech hours.

MTM is a service pharmacists provide that optimizes therapeutic outcomes for individual patients. Such services include medication therapy reviews, pharmacotherapy consults, anticoagulation management, immunizations, health and wellness programs, and many other clinical services. Pharmacists provide medication therapy management to help patients get the most benefit from their medications by actively managing drug therapy and by identifying, preventing, and resolving medication-related problems. [12]

Then, just when it seemed things could not get worse, Obamacare passed into law. The United States was now among those countries with a socialized health care system, and we did so at the cost of billions, and even trillions of dollars. Entire books have been written on this subject matter, so all I will say here is just look at Great Britain, Canada, or anywhere else where this system has been in practice for a while. In the 1960's, Claude Castonguay "the father of Quebec Medicare" chaired a Canadian government committee studying health reform, and, at the time, pushed for a government controlled healthcare system. By 2008, he admitted himself that the healthcare system he promoted was "in crisis." Similarly, Dr. Anne Doig, the Canadian Medical Association president, characterized the Canadian healthcare system as "sick" and "imploding."

---

11   http://www.cnn.com/2003/ALLPOLITICS/12/08/elec04.medicare/

12   http://www.pharmacist.com/AM/Template.cfm?section=MTM#nogo

Sally C. Pipes, President and Chief Executive Officer of the Pacific Research Institute, evaluates the massive healthcare bill passed by the Democrat controlled Congress in 2010 in her book titled The Truth About Obamacare. According to Dr. Pipes, Obamacare, "...is the largest expansion of government in the history of the United States." She goes on to describe it as, "A veritable mountain of parchment (setting) a new world record for bureaucratic overkill." She states, "Make no mistake, Obamacare will crash into our economy and culture with a tidal wave of regulations that...will fundamentally alter the way we live..." She describes how this massive government grab of one-sixth of our economy will help by, "... forcing Americans to purchase insurance," and will fine "those who refuse." She also says that, "Businesses will be coerced into providing insurance to their employees, and will be fined if they don't."

So how will Obamacare affect Medicaid? Well, according to Dr. Pipes, "Medicaid will be dramatically expanded to cover 18 million of the additional 34 million people who will now be insured." She describes Medicaid as, "One of the most financially unstable and ineffective programs of our government," and that, "Now it will grow exponentially." For a more in depth look at my opinion of Medicaid see the appendix. (Appendix J)

She's not done there. Included in her evaluation of Obamacare she states that now it, "...will also massively increase regulation of the insurance market," and will enable the government to, "...dictate to insurance companies what they must include in their coverage... and how much they must spend on claims."

The funny part is that Obama promised that this would, in the end, lower costs. Dr. Pipes wonders how that is possible when one considers that these changes will, "...require a huge new bureaucracy of administrators, regulators, consultants, and enforcement experts," for a grand total of, "159 new boards and commissions." Enforcement experts would be those in charge of compliance, keeping taxpayers in line and penalizing them if they don't cooperate, riding the backs of insurance companies, etc. Even funnier, not only did the Congressional Budget Office admit that by 2019, 23 million people will remain uninsured, but the Health and Human Services Department admitted that Obamacare would actually increase the country's overall health care bill.[13]

A cursory examination would force one to wonder why in the world would we want to implement this disastrous system. I, for one, hope this is repealed by a Republican Congress in the next few years. I mean think about it, if socialized medicine is so wonderful then why did Danny Williams, the premier of Newfoundland, travel to Miami, FL for heart surgery? Why did Belinda Stonach, liberal member of parliament, travel to California for her breast cancer operation? An entire book could be written on people, including many world leaders, who have come here to the U.S. for their medical treatment.

Let me make one thing very clear, there is no such thing as "free" healthcare. Medicaid for example is certainly not free, and it is not "insurance." It is welfare plain and simple. When a country adopts socialized healthcare, all they are doing is putting the money and power into the hands of government bureaucrats so that they can take from one group and give to another.

All one has to do is look to our neighbor to the north, America Junior, to see what is in store for us. In 2009, in Canada, 694,161 people were on waiting lists for surgery and various other necessary medical treatments. The wait time between referral and actual treatment was over 16 weeks. This is according to a 2009 report titled, "Waiting Your Turn," Hospital Waiting Lists In Canada.

In fact, according to the Organization for Economic Cooperation and Development, Canada ranks twenty-sixth out of thirty countries for number of doctors per one thousand people. When Canada first adopted Castonguay's plan, they were ranked fourth. They have dropped steadily ever since. According to Dr. Pipes, over ten percent of Canadian doctors have moved to the United States most likely due to the fact that they earn only 42 percent of what American doctors earn on average.

13   Associated Press, "Report: Health overhaul will increase USA's tab."

Great Britain is another poster child for government incompetence when it comes to running healthcare. According to an article written in Daily Mail by Jenny Hope and Nick McDermott titled, "The babies born in hospitals: Bed shortages force 4,000 mothers to give birth in lifts, offices and hospital toilets," in 2008 there were 4,000 cases of pregnant women in British hospitals who ended up having to give birth in places other than a maternity ward. Dr. Pipes writes about how in Sweden things are so bad that, "...some patients stuck on waiting lists have resorted to going to veterinarians..." Don't even get me started on Cuba! It may be Michael Moore's cup of tea, but I wouldn't exactly look to him for health advice.

Dr. Pipes also lists some statistics in her book in an effort to compare our pre-Obama healthcare system with that of other countries. "The (breast cancer) survival rate among American women is 83.9 percent, while Britain's is just 69.7 percent. For men with prostate cancer, the survival rate is 91.9 percent in the United States, 73.7 percent in France, and 51.1 percent in Britain. American men and women are more than 35 percent more likely to survive colon cancer than British citizens." She even quotes Robert Ohsfeldt of Texas A&M and John Schneider of the University of Iowa as finding in their research, "...that Americans who don't die in homicides or car accidents outlive people in every other Western country."

How does all of this affect pharmacy? I'm glad you asked. In her book, Dr. Pipes describes how, "British patients are often denied access to the newest lifesaving medicines because the National Health Service (NHS) considers them unnecessary." She states that the, "National Institute for Health and Clinical Effectiveness (NICE) determines which treatments the NHS should cover", and basically functions to, "...limit people's access to drugs." That sounds eerily similar to health care rationing, does it not?

Sarah Palin stirred up much controversy when she spoke of "death panels" as a component of Obamacare. Pundits and journalists attacked her and others who agreed, as being alarmists and fear mongers. One of those very same people was New York Times Op-

Ed columnist Paul Krugman; however, on November 14, 2010 as a guest on This Week with Christiane Amanpour he said, "Okay, look, Medicare is going to have to decide what it's going to pay for. And at least for starters, it's going to have to decide which medical procedures are not effective at all and should not be paid for at all." He went on to say, "Some years down the pike we're gonna get the real solution, which is gonna be a combination of death panels and sales taxes." So, here you have one of Obamacare's greatest supporters finally admitting that Palin's description was, in fact, correct.

Between the massive funds going into these government entitlement programs, the shift from techs to "central fill," the ever-increasing clinical components being added, and the continued devolution of basic civility one really has to wonder whether retail pharmacy will look recognizable in another ten years. When I graduated pharmacy school, pharmacists were in great demand. We would be offered signing bonuses, and companies would fall over one another to recruit us. As time went on, more pharmacy schools were being built and thus many more graduates. Not only did sign on bonuses vanish, but roles reversed and pharmacists found themselves having to beat down doors to get a job. Supply had finally exceeded demand.

If things continue on the path that is currently underway, there will most likely be a massive shift from retail to the clinical, and once again the supply of retail pharmacists will not be able to meet the demand. Increase in government regulation will also turn potential pharmacy students off especially when they realize things like the fact that it is much easier for an illegal alien to vote in this country's elections than it is for the average American to purchase pseudoephedrine at their local pharmacy. Then again, with central fill and an increased reliance on automation, perhaps things will balance out once and for all. I hope you have enjoyed this behind the scenes look at the world of retail pharmacy. For further glimpses into this universe please visit my blog site at www.retailpharmacypodcast. com, and look for my free podcast downloads at iTunes.

Appendix

A. How Your Pharmacy Works

I began working retail pharmacy nearly 16 years ago, and I, along with all of my friends in pharmacy, have been having the exact same arguments with people and have been continuously explaining precisely the same things during our entire careers. It seems that there is a persistent unfamiliarity among the populace concerning the inner workings of pharmacies. This is not to say that people are to blame, they simply have never been informed; that is the intention behind this article. It is only a microcosm in the vast universe of pharmacy, but it will cover a couple of the more common issues.

The question most often asked of retail pharmacists is what the cost of the prescription will be. Please read carefully because this is important- we can only give you the cash price of the medication before we fill it. If you have insurance, then we cannot tell you the price until we actually fill the prescription. We first have to enter your personal information including your prescription insurance info into our computer, we then type the prescription into our computer, our computer electronically transmits your prescription to your insurance company's computer, which then processes the prescription and transmits the price that we are to charge you to our printer. Only at this point do we know the cost to you, but it takes times as you can see, and we have not even physically filled the prescription yet. Prescription insurance companies are the main reason for your extended wait times.

Now, if upon hearing the cost you feel that it is incorrect, then you need to contact your prescription insurance company. Remember, they are sending the cost to you- to us. We have essentially no say in what you get charged. Simply call the 1-800 number on the back of your card and they will be able to directly answer all of your questions; they can even give you the price before you go to the pharmacy. Again, they set the price, not us.

You may have heard the words "prior authorization" at the pharmacy at some point or another. This is the latest trend in third party over-stepping. Basically what your prescription insurance company is saying is that despite the fact that your doctor wrote the prescription him or herself, they still require that he or she call them on the phone and authorize it. If that does not seem to make any sense to you, do not fret for it does not make much sense to us either. What we do is call the doctor's office, tell them we need a "prior auth", give them your insurance's phone number, and then wait for them to call us back with the authorization so that we can transmit your prescription through the insurance. It sounds like a blast doesn't it?

Communication is a crucial component of the pharmacist-patient relationship. Whether a patient is dropping off or picking up a prescription, the pharmacist may need to speak to him or her, and ask or answer certain questions. The laws governing a person's health information have gotten stricter since HIPPA took effect in 2003. It stipulates what we are permitted to do with your personal health info, and what we are not permitted to do. We are legally responsible for your privacy, and cannot have others hearing what we are saying to you about your health care information.

Patients who come up to our windows gabbing away on a cell phone are preventing us from being able to abide by the HIPPA laws. It also makes it extremely difficult to counsel patients on their drugs (i.e., dosage, side effects, drug interactions, etc.). Absolutely nothing should come between a pharmacist and the patient's safety, so please hang up.

What ever happened to common courtesy and social etiquette? How have we regressed to the point where now the average person can be so oblivious in their daily interactions so as to not even realize how staggeringly impolite it is to yammer away on a phone while trying to solicit a retail transaction. The lack of even an inkling of awareness, or a rudimentary sense of shame in these people is astonishing. The fact that it just might be inappropriate to do such a foolish thing never dawns upon them. To these people I plead 'help us to help you'.

On behalf of all pharmacists, pharmacy technicians, and retail clerks in general, please use some common sense and self-awareness, and get off of the phone before you walk up to our windows or cash registers. It would be prudent to say the least. In the name of politeness, courtesy, and, in our case regard for safety, please give us your undivided attention. Your health may depend upon it.

B. Advice For Snowbirds

In Southwest Florida "season" has arrived and that means that the snowbirds have migrated back to Florida. This particular group of people provides special challenges for local residents and workers, and retail pharmacists are no exception. One attribute that seems to be universal among snowbirds (besides rudeness) is impatience. Everyone, by now, is enjoying the trench warfare-like process of seeing a cascade of patients. During season, wait times for prescriptions are generally much longer because we are much busier than usual, hence the aforementioned designation. Medical professionals look forward to this time of year about as much as the boys eying the beaches of Normandy just before the ramps lowered. What follows are only a few small requests on behalf of the pharmacy world.

Doctors, please take the extra 2.3 seconds it takes to write a tad more legibly. I could put a pen in a parakeet's claw, and get scratchings more closely resembling letters and words. Often times, after staring at a prescription for eight solid minutes, I begin to feel like Russell Crowe in a Beautiful Mind convinced that there is some hidden message on the paper before me, and am determined to decipher it.

Nurses also need to write a little clearer, but it is in this regard only that they excel over the parakeet. For now, let's focus on the calling in of prescriptions to our automated answering service. Most nurses, ostensibly because they are very busy, speak faster than a meth addict on his 6th cappa-frappa-latte-whatever when calling in a prescription. Ladies, please slow it down to about 125 rpms, okay?

Secondly, I beg you, for the love of almighty God, spell the doctor's name. You spell the patient's name about 50% of the time, but with eerie consistency, almost never spell the doctor's name. You see, we do not work with this person all day long as you do, and so their name is not as familiar to us. All we ask is a little common sense. If the M.D.'s name is "Doctor Supercalifragilistics", then you may want to spell it for us, all right? The bizarre and amazing consistency with which this is not done makes me think that there is a massive conspiracy here just waiting to be exposed. Forget Lochness, Big Foot, J.F.K., the moon landing, etc., this nurse-non-spelling-the-doctor's-name thing could be just about the largest scandal in all of history!

Lastly, patients please be patient. We realize that you are not feeling particularly well, otherwise you would not be coming to visit us. We will fill your prescription as quickly as we can, but try to remember...all of those other people that you see standing all around you glaring at us, as you are, are also waiting for their prescription. If you are standing behind them, then that means that they were here first. Are you beginning to get the picture now? Also, please be civil. "Why are you yelling at me?" is a question I ought not have to ask. Now, if we do not seem to be as sunny and cheerful as you require, then we apologize, but try to keep in mind that we have been stuck in this tiny room for over 12 hours with barely a bathroom break, with no food break, and with people literally screaming at us all day long. It tends to wear a person down.

Common among snowbirds is either forgetting to bring the prescription insurance card south, or the drugs themselves. Here is some advice that all pharmacy patients can benefit from- without the card, it is nearly impossible to run the prescription through your insurance properly. There are numbers that only pharmacists use, and certain logos or insignia that tip us off to the intricacies of your particular insurance coverage. The bottom line is that you must bring your card with you for any first time visit. Once it is in the computer, then you need not present it again. We are able to call your insurance company, or northern pharmacy, and get the necessary information, but this adds significantly to your wait time.

Something else to remember is the fact that each state has it's own set of pharmacy laws, and those laws do tend to change from time to time. Every pharmacist has heard, "My pharmacy back home was able to do it!" or "You did it last time!" As much as we may wish to help you, we cannot break the law. Why customers would rather yell and argue as opposed to trust our word for something is vexing. Hint: yelling at us does not change the law, or our duty to abide by it.

No doubt, by now you are beginning to develop a deep appreciation for the complications and intricacies inherent in pharmacy operations. These tidbits will hopefully help snowbirds, and others, overcome their trials and tribulations at the pharmacy counter much more easily during season. One last piece of advice for our semi-annual friends- left lane fast, right lane slow, okay? Got that? And we thank you. Oh yes, and welcome back to Florida!

C. Pharmacy Practice In Florida

I worked in a retail pharmacy in Orlando, Florida for five years, and came across many problems due to the vast influx of illegal immigrants into the state. Communication with people who do not speak English is an increasing problem in states like Florida, Texas, Arizona, and California. The new emphasis on patient care in the field of pharmacy means that communication is quickly becoming the most important aspect of a pharmacist's responsibilities. When confronted by a language barrier, matters drastically become complicated, and can impede a pharmacist from being as effective as they otherwise would be.

How do you properly counsel a patient on their medications when they cannot understand a word you are saying? This is a problem I had to face all day long in the pharmacy where I worked. We implemented a few strategies to combat this. One thing we did was to have a sheet of Spanish phrases that we would commonly use in our pharmacy. For instance, at our fingertips we had the Spanish equivalents for "Take once a day", "Call your doctor if you have any problems", "How do you feel?", "Where does it hurt?", etc. We were unable to carry out a complete conversation, but this did help in the patient's understanding of how to properly take their medications and what to do if there were any problems, and it helped in our understanding of their specific problems as well.

Another tactic employed by our company was to hire Spanish-speaking pharmacists and technicians. Communication, of course, became much easier; however, I have personal reservations concerning this. First, this does not provide any incentive for Hispanics to learn how to speak English. Secondly, these patients would only come to get their prescriptions filled if the Spanish speaking person was working. Thirdly, once word got out, then droves of Hispanic patients would come into our pharmacy and overload our Hispanic pharmacist whenever he was working. Many people came just to socialize. This prevented the pharmacist from focusing attention on more important matters. Lastly, we non-Spanish speaking people were left out of all conversations, and had no idea what exactly was being said; we were unable to help and felt useless. It seemed awfully rude to us as well.

Our company would also post bilingual signs, and all of our OTC and HBA products were printed in Spanish and English. Once again, I have personal problems with this. In my opinion, English ought to be the official language of America, and anyone coming here ought to be courteous enough to learn it. Catering to them only eliminates their incentive to learn English. I do not want to see us become like Canada where all signs are bilingual (French & English) because it removes any sense of national unity and identity. Being forced to speak Spanish, in my opinion, defeats the purpose of being born American.

There are also programs and classes set up specifically for pharmacists who desire to learn Spanish in order to better communicate with their consumer base. The Hispanic population is growing exponentially in this country, and the influx is beginning to spread further and further north affecting many states besides just the border states. These classes may not be a bad idea for pharmacists who work in heavily populated Hispanic communities.

My personal favorite method of communicating with Hispanic customers is through their family or friends who speak English, and can translate for them. Talking through an interpreter is a slow process, but at least it shows that they are willing to make an effort to help not only the pharmacy staff, but themselves as well. I get particularly perturbed when Hispanic customers actually get angry because we do not speak their language. It takes some nerve to come to a foreign country and demand that they speak your language, and then become upset when they do not! This is where the entitlement mentality has brought us in this country.

I periodically worked in a retail pharmacy very close to Disney World in Orlando. We would have foreigners from all over the world in our store. All of them spoke English. It seems, for some reason, that only the Hispanics refuse to speak it. Once again, it is because we cater to them and remove the incentive to learn our language. There are no signs in French, German, Chinese, Japanese, or any other language. It is because of their sheer numbers that businesses cater to them. Greed is good in many ways, but this is one example where principle ought to supersede the need to make a buck.

Once their children assimilate, then things will improve. Most Hispanic children can speak English. Also, their last names will change as they marry into our culture. This will be a huge benefit for pharmacies because Spanish last names are also a big issue. First of all, they do not really have last names in their culture. It is hard to explain, but they really do not designate last names like we do here in the U.S. Trying to find a prescription for a Spanish person is very difficult if you have to ask them what their last name is.

Another problem is that even if they have designated a "last" name for themselves, they all pick from an extremely limited list of choices. When 75% of your customers all have the last name "Rodriguez" or "Martinez", then it makes it hard to find the proper prescription. Also, their first names are not varied much either. Most women are "Maria" and most men are "Jose". It is amazing how many different customers are named Jose Rodriguez, or Maria Martinez. They make John Smith and Sally Jones look like Keir Van Damme and Natasha Lipinski.

Reflexively irate and overly sensitive politically correct, knee-jerk liberals may consider these to be harsh comments, but they are merely an accurate interpretation made by a completely honest person with first-hand experience. Opinions vary, but the facts are undeniable. I would never treat any foreigner poorly just because they are foreign. It is my duty to do everything I can to help my patients get the best care possible. The onus lies mainly with the pharmacist, but there are limits. One example is being required to learn a completely new language. This rant is moot, however, because the problem is too out of control right now for hopes of a short-term cure. In time, as assimilation occurs, things will become easier not just for pharmacists, but for Hispanic patients as well.

D. Where Should the Onus Be?

Who has not heard the expression, "the customer is always right"? This seems like a great idea for the business world where it is imperative to coddle consumers so as to make them repeat customers. For those of you who have worked retail before, particularly a retail pharmacy, you know how this principle can be abused by certain customers/patients who try to take it to the nth degree.

We all know, or should by now, that being a pharmacist involves a great deal of responsibility. I'm not just talking about the obvious responsibilities of checking for drug interactions, watching for contraindications, or resolving third party conflicts. One issue becoming more prevalent all the time is the process of communicating with patients and making sure they understand everything about their medications that they need to in order to provide them the best patient care possible. What happens, as is becoming more prevalent nowadays, when your customer base consists of patients from diverse backgrounds? How can you, as a pharmacist, best serve your patients when they come from so many different cultures, speak various languages, and hold many different beliefs and values from your own? Is it better to try to treat each and every patient as a separate individual and account for all of their idiosyncrasies, or would it be more efficient to treat all of your patients in basically the same manner and let them adapt to you?

The knee-jerk response of compassion, very prevalent in America today, may lead one to immediately say that the pharmacist should do his or her best to deal with each patient on an individual basis. The argument is that in order to provide the best patient care the pharmacist must try to be aware of different ideologies and beliefs held by people of different backgrounds so as to avoid offending them. In some cultures, for example, it is rude to look someone in the eye that is older than yourself. Some cultures have very strong beliefs about medicine and healing that may be very different from anything a student would learn in an American pharmacy school. This would mean that the pharmacist, in addition to what he or she learned in school, would have to also learn what people of different ethnicities think about medicine and healing. Some cultures, for example, put a lot more faith in herbal medications than we do here in America. This reasoning would result in the pharmacist having to be aware of these differences in case anyone from a particular culture should happen to bring a prescription in to be filled.

The other side of the argument states that perhaps it would be better if the pharmacist or technician just stay constant, and treat patients in the same manner. If special circumstances are required for someone who does not speak the language, for example, they can take the initiative and bring in someone, a friend or family member, who speaks English and can translate for them. Advocates of this point of view may argue that there is just too much variety out there and it is ludicrous to expect a pharmacist, or anyone working retail, to cater to everyone who walks into their store. Perhaps foreigners coming into the pharmacy who are from another culture could try to realize on their own that any offense by a pharmacist or technician is purely accidental, not intentional. Maybe they could use a little foresight and realize that there are many different ethnicities to account for in this country and that misunderstandings are inevitable.

It is interesting how the responsibility is always placed on the server and not the one being served. Pharmacy, which is basically the only health profession that exists in a retail environment, is especially interesting because one would think that, when it comes to health, the one being served would do their best to makes things as easy for the pharmacist as possible. The opposite seems to be true, however.

Not only is the pharmacist expected to perform his or her normal responsibilities as quickly as possible and with no errors, but now it seems as though he or she is also expected to know every subtle nuance that exists in the world and be an international translator as well. This is just one example of how attitudes are changing around the world and especially in this country. Everyone is so paranoid about offending someone else and those who get offended seem to do so over the most inane things. Touchiness has reached a new plateau and it has resulted in making life much more difficult than it needs to be. God forbid anyone should say or do something that offends someone else. Unless we all start to relax a little and quit taking trivial things so seriously, matters are going to get a lot worse.

E. Pharmacy Rules of Conduct

Be on time (if not, be sure to call), and be ready to work when you punch in.

Acknowledge person at the counter as soon as they walk up (if busy say, "I'll be right there" or "I'll be right with you", etc.). Do not make them wait too long. Always be kind, courteous, and polite.

When a patient is dropping off a rx, always make sure that their name, the Dr.'s name, and the name of the drug are legible. Also, write the patient's date of birth on the rx.

At pick up, always make sure you have the correct patient vis-à-vis their date of birth, address, etc., the number of rxs they are picking up, and for notes left by the pharmacist on the bag.

Never tell the pharmacist to get the window. If someone walks up behind the person you're helping, then just say, "I'll be right with you." If the patient has a question, inform them that you will have the pharmacist come over at his earliest convenience. Do not ask from across the pharmacy, and immediately interrupt the pharmacist, especially if he or she is in the middle of doing something. Do not stand hovering over us waiting. Write down your question if you're afraid you may forget.

Rescue the pharmacist from the register if possible, especially during season.

If a patient wants a transfer, but does not have their bottle, we need - name and phone number of pharmacy where rx currently is, the patient's name, date of birth, and drug name. Always check to see if refills remain, and inform pharmacist if it is a controlled drug. All transfers are 24 hours during season.

Salvage anything that can be used repeatedly. No reason why we cannot use bags, vials that have never left the pharmacy, "refrigerate" or "mixing" notes, etc.

Multitask. There is no reason why you cannot be on hold with an insurance and type another rx at the same time, or ring up a customer.

The phone should not ring more than twice. If you are busy, then answer it and ask them if you may place them on hold.

When putting the order away, always place new drugs behind the old ones on the shelf, and always place in alphabetical order. If you're not sure where something goes, please ask. There is no guessing in pharmacy.

Always place the patient's bags in proper alphabetical order in the "Will Call Bin."

At any time, if you notice multiple bags for a single patient in the bins, then combine their bags into one. This provides more space and prevents waste.

Check NDC # when pulling bottles off of the shelf. It's better to pull the bottle off of the shelf before actually filling the script. This will save editing time.

Get rid of old manufacturer's drug bottles first. They will expire first.

"X" a bottle when you open it, and do not open multiple bottles of the same drug.

Three waiters at a time maximum, and be sure to properly indicate which are.

If a patient has more than one profile, choose the most recently used one; merge if possible. If the M.D. has more than one, then chose the one with most current phone number. If the phone number is outdated, then please update in the computer. If the patient's insurance is no longer valid, then deactivate it.

For CII scripts, check for correct NDC # and quantity (via the CII book) before the patient leaves & before typing. The pharmacist may have to help you here.

If you are not absolutely positive about what a rx says, then ask the pharmacist or call the M.D. No assumptions.

Many sigs are written on two lines. Be sure to type both.

Try to be quick, but not at the expense of accuracy.

If ordering a drug for a patient, tell them it will be in on the promised day at 4 PM.

Watch quantities when filling a rx. Sometimes omeprazole 40mg is for #60 (two bottles) or albuterol inhaler is for a quantity of 34 (two inhalers), etc.

If a suspension is written for quantity 50 mL, and it only comes as 60 mL, we must fill for a quantity of 60 mL.

Always edit and correct a wrong NDC # when filling.

When filling rxs, separate patients from one another, and group multiple rxs for a single patient together. This will prevent possible bagging of rxs for two different people in the same bag. It also prevents multiple bagging of a single patient's rxs.

Watch rx stickers! Do not place "pregnancy" stickers on rxs for males, or women too young or too old. No "alcohol" or "driving" stickers for children. Etc.

Staple insurance rejections to the bag. Rather than take our word for it, we can show the patient exactly what the rejection says, and they can see it for themselves.

Watch what you are throwing away. Sometimes it is an insurance rejection, or something else that we need.

Check the queue frequently (every 10 or 15 minutes) to see if new rxs are waiting to be filled. Periodically check printer too to see if printed rxs are waiting to be filled.

When organizing rxs into California folders, make sure they are all the same kind before shelving them (i.e., no control rxs ought to be in a Calif. folder with regular scripts and vice versa), and place in numerical order.

All techs are responsible for the basic tech duties. No one is above running the register, taking out the trash, stocking supplies, etc.

We should never run out of supplies, especially during season. If anyone notices that a supply is getting dangerously low, then leave a note so that it may be ordered. If a drug is getting low, especially a fast mover, then add it to that evening's order manually.

Please let the pharmacist know when you go on break or leave the pharmacy.

Finish tasks, do not leave for the next day unless completely unavoidable.

No cell phones, and please limit personal calls/visits, especially during busy hours.

30 days notice for vacation requests. 14 days for general time off requests. Techs requesting a day off before these deadlines must find another trained tech to fill in for them, not a cashier.

Your schedule and weekly hours are always subject to change.

F. My Letter to the Florida Pharmacy Association (2007)

Dear Mr. Jackson,

My name is Jean-Marc Bovee, Pharm.D., and I have a concern that has worried me for many years now, and continues to grow more urgent in my mind. I have worked in the retail pharmacy world as a technician and as a pharmacist for over 15 years now, and what troubles me more and more, and has motivated me to contact you, is the quality, or should I say poor quality, of pharmacy technicians in the state of Florida.

Before I go any further I feel the need to state that I am not an egotist who looks down on pharmacy technicians as so many R.Ph.s do. I was a tech myself for many years before even being accepted to pharmacy school. I have been a personal friend with many of the techs I have worked with. My brother is presently a pharmacy technician.

Having said that, what worries me is how many pharmacy technicians are so very unqualified to work behind a pharmacy counter that I fear not only for my license on a daily basis, but also for my patient's safety. The fact that this is not yet an epidemic being reported in the media is a testament I feel to the unbelievable job R.Ph.s everywhere are doing to curtail this problem. However, if something is not done soon either in Tallahassee, or better yet Washington D.C., then this will inevitably be a story splattered all over the news media. That 20/20 story on pharmacy errors a few months back was just the tip of the iceberg, and a warning call for all of us.

I have worked for four major companies as well as an independent pharmacy in three major cities in two different states. In Orlando alone, as a technician seeking overtime to get through school at UCF, I worked in over half-a-dozen different pharmacies with over 20 different pharmacists and even more technicians. I know the retail pharmacy world like the back of my hand. I have never been fired; dangerous technicians dug in like tics was the primary motivation for these moves, as well as finance. I say all of this so that you will know where I am coming from. I am telling you that over 60% of the pharmacy technicians that I have worked with during my career are dangerously unqualified, and I use the word dangerously literally.

Let me ask you a few questions: Is there any other branch of medicine where anyone off of the street can be hired and begin working intimately in the medical setting like pharmacy technicians can? Is there any other branch of medicine where the support staff (i.e., dental assistants, physician assistants, nurses, etc.) is not required to have some sort of standardized training or certification? The time has come for this in pharmacy.

Let me ask you a few more questions: Do you think a technician ought to be able to multiply 7 X 6 without asking for the answer? Do you think a technician ought to know what "AD" means in a sig? Do you think a pharmacy technician ought to be able to subtract 13 from 100 without using a calculator? Do you think that the average pharmacy technician ought to be able to add allergies to a patient's profile? Sir, these are real life situations that occurred in my pharmacy with my technician YESTERDAY, and have prompted me to write to you. This sort of thing occurs in my pharmacy every single day, and this technician is not the first by a long shot. As I said, 60% of the ones I have seen are positively lethal.

By the way, this technician has 20 years experience as a pharmacy technician with the company that I presently work for, and 10 years before that working for an independent pharmacy. You read that correctly...30 years experience.

I hope you will contact me to discuss this matter further.

239-XXX-XXXX

I personally am ready to do whatever it takes to convince the state, and the nation, to pass mandatory training and certification requirements for pharmacy technicians. I will lobby Tallahassee, Washington D.C., whomever I must because this has to stop. If things do not change, then may God have mercy on our patients. If you think I am being melodramatic, then allow me to point out that I am not a religious man, but yet I humbly beg for help.

Sincerely,

Jean-Marc Bovee

Dear Dr. Bovee,

The issue of credentialing pharmacist technicians is of particular interest within the Florida Pharmacy Association. Our Association, as with the members of the Florida Society of Health Systems Pharmacists agree that there is a need for regulations defining the qualification and educational standards of pharmacy supportive personnel. There are currently two bills that have been filed for consideration by the Florida legislature on this issue. While these bills are a start there is some work that needs to be done on the proposals. The FPA Legislative Committee met this summer and has placed in as an action plan to work with FSHP on the passage of a bill that would require pharmacist technician registration and certification.

Currently in Florida the "minimum" requirements for an individual to serve as a pharmacist technician is to be able to wear a name badge that says "pharmacist technician". With that designation an individual can assist the pharmacist with nearly all aspects of the prescription dispensing process that does not require professional judgment. Pharmacist technicians in Florida can also initiate and receive communication from the prescriber's office on refill authorizations provided that there is not a change in therapy.

It is important to note that on the prescriber side there are no requirements for training for individuals who transmit prescription information to the pharmacy which makes it doubly important for someone on the receiving end of a called in prescription to be qualified, certified and trained. Of course the designation dental assistants, physician assistants and other midlevel practitioners require education, training and credentialing. Also there are many technicians assisting Florida licensed pharmacists that are very good at what they do and are an essential part of the pharmacy health care team. Florida has nearly 13,000 certified pharmacy technicians. Texas and California are the only state with more. It is time that those individuals become recognized for their contribution to health care.

Pharmacist duties and responsibilities have extended into drug therapy management programs. We are finding that there is considerable interest in expanding or removing pharmacist to technician ratios. Such efforts to do so should not occur without some review and consideration for the qualifications and training of all individuals involved in the management of patient prescription drug therapy.

The Florida Pharmacy Association has scheduled a Legislative Day in Tallahassee on March 5, 2008 with a Health Fair on March 6th. You may want to look at your schedule to see if you are able to participate. If you have others in your pharmacy community that are interested they are welcome to participate as well.

I have copied your concerns with the FPA Legislative Committee and hope that you do not mind.

Michael A. J------, R.CPh.
Executive Vice President and CEO
Florida Pharmacy Association
Tallahassee, Florida 32301
www.pharmview.com
(850) XXX-XXXX

G. Oxycodone

Perhaps the most worrisome of all retail pharmacy customers are those coming in asking for oxycodone, which is a very potent and addictive painkiller. Pharmacies, especially in the state of Florida, are increasingly being inundated by "oxy seekers" to the point where hardly a day can go by without some doctor having their license suspended for over-prescribing, a newspaper article discussing some sort of assault and arrest, or a pharmacy being robbed concerning this drug.

In 2009, a report by The Florida Medical Examiners Commission showed that far more people die from prescription drug use than illicit drug use, and oxycodone was responsible for 1,185 Floridian deaths - more any other type of drug. Florida lacks any form of regulation over pain clinics also known as "pill mills" that profit from prescribing painkillers indiscriminately. The pills can then be sold on the street at ten times the cost. [14] These institutions are popping up all over Florida at a geometric rate.

Fortunately, people seeking oxycodone are not very imaginative or nuanced. In fact, they are easier to spot than Barack Obama's ears. First of all they all smell like chain smokers, and if you get close enough, booze too. Secondly, they all look like they had staring rolls in Idiocracy. If that doesn't help, then just think – Rob Zombie. Thirdly, and this comes in handy when they call your pharmacy, they all have the same melodious vocal tones of Jason Mewes.

For the most part, pharmacists either do not keep the drug in stock, or they only fill prescriptions for their regular customers; the ones who actually need it. Understandably, pharmacy supervisors and their superiors insist and demand that pharmacists keep a regular supply on hand at all times. Thus, each individual pharmacist must make a professional judgment as when to fill oxycodone prescriptions and when not to.

This puts them in a precarious situation because if a prescription is filled for some doctor-shopper type who winds up selling these drugs on the street, then the pharmacist who filled it can be just as liable as the doctor who wrote it. My advice is to err on the side of caution, and not to fill if the person seems disreputable. It is better to get fired than to be arrested. After all, it is the pharmacist who fills the prescription whose medical license is at stake, not his or her supervisor's.

14   http://charlotte.floridaweekly.com/news/2010-07-08/Top_News/
WARNING_May_Cause_Addiction.html

H.

Daily Closing Duties

- Fill vials and caps
- Fill printer and fax machine
- Fill rx bags and staplers
- Check supplies and order if needed
- Empty trash and shredder
- Organize paper prescriptions (sticker and place in order in Calif. folder)
- Hang filled rxs in Will Call Bin
- Vacuum and dust if needed

Daily Opening Duties

- Get register money from cash office
- Make Dr. calls (refills, prior auths, etc.)
- Complete Fill queue
- Reverse prescriptions 10 days old and older and return to stock.
- Check in orders and complete Fill On Arrival
- Help other stores with Data Entry

I.

Attention Floaters

The following is a reminder of your duties and our expectations for you when filling in at stores, particularly where there are no technicians available. Pharmacist, as well as patient complaints, renders this memo necessary.

1. Be courteous to the customers. Remember, they are regulars at this store.

2. Sign in on Dispensing Record Logbook.

3. Please make all 7-day calls & do 10-day returns.

4. Please check in all orders, and complete the paperwork.

5. If CIIs come in, check in the order and log into the CII book as well.

6. Please do not reorganize the pharmacy. Be neat and clean. Leave it as you   found it.

7. Do all recalls on the WIRE for that day.

8. If no tech is present, then please perform closing duties- take out trash, fill printer, caps, vials, etc., and sticker the filled rxs for the day.

9. Take register money to cash office at the end of the night.

10. Please leave your contact information in case someone needs to follow up with you on something.

J. Medicaid Is Not Free

Working retail pharmacy allows for the ability to see and hear some startling things, and some just continue to worsen. One is the growing misconception that Medicaid provides free stuff. Lately, it has been said to me that "Medicaid is great because it's free", and, after inquiring about the cash price of a medication, one lady who boasted that she has been on Medicaid for 16 years said, "Nope, let Medicaid pay for it."

Something needs to be explained. Medicaid is not free; taxpayers fund it. It is the pharmacist, the pharmacy technician, the cashier, the grocery bagger, and every other hard working person who is paying for it. According to the Florida Pharmacy Association, $15.3 billion, or about 25%, of the state's annual budget is devoted to Medicaid. In 1998 it was $800 million. By 2015, it will consume 60% of the state budget. It cannot be said enough; these are taxpayer's dollars being used. This is what led to the passage of Proposition 187 in California that prohibits illegal immigrants from receiving most public benefits. Following are more statistics on the issue.

In a 1994 article titled Illegal Immigrants Abuse Health Care Services, Gayle Hanson explains that since the passage of the 1986 Omnibus Budget Reconciliation Act, which "requires states to provide emergency medical and childbirth services to all illegal immigrants through Medicaid programs, the number of people taking advantage of free medical care has grown eighteen fold." This was 11 years ago. She also stated that, "…40% of all publicly funded births are to illegal immigrants," and that, "…many of the services provided to undocumented immigrants…are not available to legal residents."

Sally Super, who was the director of the maternity pavilion at Sharp Chula Vista Hospital at the time, stated, "We have women coming here and they only know how to say two things in English. They want a birth certificate and they want to know how to apply for the Women Infants and Children (WIC) Program." She also complained that she and her staff were not even allowed to inquire about their legal status.

A 1995 article by Donald Huddle titled Illegal Immigrants Are an Economic Burden lists what benefits illegals are entitled to, "…food stamps, housing assistance, WIC, unemployment compensation, job training, Medicaid, the earned income tax credit," etc.

A study tilted The High Cost of Cheap Labor, Illegal Immigration and the Federal Budget estimated the total impact of illegal immigration on the federal budget. Among the findings: households headed by illegal aliens imposed more than $26.3 billion in costs on the federal government in 2002 and paid only $16 billion in taxes, creating a net fiscal deficit of almost $10.4 billion. The single largest cost was Medicaid ($2.5 billion).

In August 2002 an inspector general's report found that most states do not verify claims of U.S. citizenship by those applying for Medicaid benefits. Only Montana, New York, New Hampshire and Texas require applicants to submit documents verifying citizenship. Of the states that allow self-declaration of citizenship before accessing Medicaid, 27 did not conduct subsequent auditing that would verify an applicant's statements to be true. Only one state, Oregon, has conducted an audit to determine how often "non-citizens" gained access to Medicaid.

In an August 10, 2005 article titled Medicaid Fraud the Apparent Price for Cutting Red Tape by Alexa Moutevelis, she presents a U.S. Justice Department report showing that 47 states allow Medicaid applicants to vouch for their own legal U.S. citizenship when applying for benefits, and more than half of those states do not follow up in trying to verify the self-declarations. Jack Martin, special projects director for the Federation for American Immigration Reform (FAIR), admits that, "there's basically no way to know how many people are getting Medicaid illegally."

According to the report issued by the Justice Department's Office of the Inspector General, illegal immigrants have been encouraged to declare their citizenship status in order to simplify the Medicaid applications. John Valentine, CEO of InfoGlide, when asked to rank the fraud types, commented, "…the big one is Medicaid. Many states could buy an NFL football team with what they could save in Medicaid fraud - each year."

In the Spring 2005 edition of the Journal of American Physicians and Surgeons, Madeleine Cosman, Ph.D., Esq. wrote an article titled Illegal Aliens and American Medicine where she states such things as the fact that between 1993 and 2003, 60 California hospitals went bankrupt and closed down due to the influx of illegal immigrants, and 70% of babies born in San Joaquin General Hospital in Stockton, California were those of non-citizens. She shows that Medicaid actually provides illegal aliens with translators, and MediCal in 2003 had 760,000 illegals signed up. She states bluntly that, "Scams, frauds, and cheats are rampant." (sources: 1994 U.S. House of Representatives, Committee on Ways and Means, Subcommittee on Oversight report; testimony by the Senate Appropriations Committee, Subcommittee on Labor, HHS, and Education; 2004 L.A., California Center for the Study of Popular Culture report; etc.).

The abuse of Medicaid and other welfare programs by illegal aliens has been thoroughly documented all over our country. The evidence is there for those concerned about this misappropriation of tax dollars. We can no longer allow political parties to buy votes with our tax dollars. Especially when the money that goes into these entitlement programs comes from American citizens who these programs were meant to help in the first place.

The people of each state must address this issue in the same way the people of California did vis-à-vis Proposition 187. If this concerns you, then write your representatives in congress and voice your objections. If you still do not believe this is a serious problem, then ask any pharmacist whether they believe it is more difficult for an illegal alien to vote in this country's elections, or for an American citizen to purchase pseudoephedrine? We simply can no longer afford to give so many people a free ride.

Glossary

1. Tech- a pharmacy technician; someone who assists the pharmacist in performing his or her duties.

2. RX- a prescription; an instruction written by a medical practitioner

3. IVR- interactive voice response; basically a pharmacy answering machine where doctors, nurses, or patients can leave messages for the pharmacist.

4. QRE- Quality Related Event; in other words, an error committed in the pharmacy on a prescription.

5. PITA- Pain In The Ass

6. OTC- over the counter; any medication not requiring a prescription

7. Oxy seeker- typically young Caucasian male in his mid twenties wearing baggy pants and a baseball cap sporting multiple tattoos and piercings wreaking of cigarettes who acts likes a pharmacist's best friend so that he can

get his oxycodone 15mg, 30mg, and alprazolam 2mg prescriptions filled because the sell for a bundle per tablet on the street.

8. Pill Mill- a doctor's office, clinic, or health care facility that prescribes controlled drugs outside the scope of prevailing standards of medical practice thus violating the law.

9. Doctor Shopper- the illegal practice of a patient requesting care from multiple physicians, often simultaneously, without making efforts to coordinate care or informing the physicians of the multiple caregivers.